Expecting Joy

A Complete Guide to a
Healthy Pregnancy

By
Well-Being Publishing

To You,

Thank you!

Table of Contents

Expecting Joy:
A Complete Guide to
a Healthy Pregnancy

Welcome to the incredible journey of pregnancy, a time that's as replete with wonder as it is with questions. As you embark on this life-changing experience, it's essential to arm yourself with knowledge that empowers you while nurturing the little life within you. Embracing a healthy pregnancy sets both you and your baby up for a thriving start.

Pregnancy is not just a physical change or a solitary process—it's a transformation that encompasses the emotional, mental, and spiritual state of an expectant mother. It's a time filled with anticipation, planning, and, most importantly, the opportunity to bond with your unborn child. This first chapter serves as your starting point, guiding you through the fundamentals of what it means to have a healthy pregnancy.

Understanding your body's transformation during pregnancy is not just fascinating; it's crucial. With each passing week, your body achieves remarkable feats to accommodate the new life growing within you. Your heart works harder, your blood volume increases, and you begin to feel the physical signs of life stirring within.

Mental well-being is just as imperative as physical health during this time. It's perfectly normal to experience a carousel of emotions—from elation to apprehension—and understanding these feelings can help you manage them. Being kind to yourself, acknowledging your emotions, and seeking support are integral parts of a joyous pregnancy experience.

Further, establishing a robust support network is invaluable. Whether it's your partner, family, or friends, having people you can turn to for reassurance and help can make all the difference. This network will be your go-to not just for practical tasks but also for the sometimes-needed emotional boost.

Preparing for your prenatal visits is another significant step in this journey. These check-ups are a window into your baby's development and your health. They also serve as a platform for asking questions and voicing any concerns. Don't hesitate to prepare a list of topics you wish to discuss with your healthcare provider beforehand.

Understanding the changes in your body, acknowledging the rollercoaster of emotions that might come, and setting up a support system all forge the path to a healthy pregnancy. Your proactive involvement in each stage will help you gain confidence and enjoyment as you near closer to meeting your little one.

One of the most profound aspects of pregnancy is witnessing your body perform its natural magic. The first fluttering sensations of your baby moving, the visible changes as your bump grows—these are all parts of the remarkable transformation your body undergoes.

While the physical signs are often the most discussed aspect of pregnancy, there's an emotional journey that goes hand-in-hand with the physical one. It's an excellent time to reflect on your hopes, discuss your fears openly, and create a vision for the kind of parent you aspire to be.

As you navigate through these shifts, remember that you're not alone on this voyage. It's not uncommon to feel overwhelmed, but there's a wealth of resources available to you—from healthcare professionals to community groups and literature dedicated to expectant parents.

Making informed choices is another cornerstone of a healthy pregnancy. Understanding the options available to you in childbirth, feeding, and caring for your newborn allows you to make decisions that align with your personal beliefs, health considerations, and lifestyle preferences.

Embracing self-care routines, such as balanced nutrition and appropriate exercise, will not only contribute to the well-being of your baby but will also enhance your overall health. This is the time to prioritize yourself, ensuring that your body has the strength and vitality it needs to nurture your growing baby.

Amidst all this preparation, don't forget to celebrate the small milestones. Each week brings you closer to the day you'll hold your baby. Taking the journey one step at a time allows you to not only focus on the present but also to anticipate the joys that await you ahead.

This guide is your companion, illuminating the path ahead with insight and warmth. While no two pregnancies are the same, there are universal truths and solid advice that can help ease the way. By integrating this knowledge into your unique journey, you're setting the stage for a healthier, happier pregnancy filled with joy and anticipation.

To conclude, this chapter sets the foundation for a deeply enriching experience during one of life's most profound transitions. As you move forward to the subsequent chapters, you'll delve into more specific aspects of pregnancy, equipped with the understanding and positivity you need to navigate this special time with grace and excitement.

Chapter 1:
Introduction

Welcome to a journey like no other. Bringing new life into the world is one of the most profound experiences you'll ever encounter, filled with wonder, challenges, transformation, and profound joy. Whether you're an expectant mother, a supportive partner, a family member brimming with excitement, a friend looking to offer support, or a healthcare professional guiding the way — this book is crafted to be your companion during one of life's most incredible adventures: pregnancy.

Pregnancy is a time of extraordinary change, not just physically but emotionally and mentally. It's a period when you're likely to have a multitude of questions and perhaps a few concerns too. That's why education and preparation are key — not just to ease worries but to empower you with knowledge and confidence. This book is designed to do just that, providing you with up-to-date information, practical advice, and empathy, ensuring you feel prepared for the many aspects of this life-changing experience.

The following pages will be an invaluable resource as you navigate the triumphs and trials of pregnancy. They'll offer expert guidance, insights into your body's incredible capabilities, and advice on how to care for both your physical and emotional wellbeing. Remember, while pregnancy is a time of great physical change, it also invites you on a profound inner journey that's to be embraced and honored.

As you progress through each trimester, you're likely to notice a magnificent display of your body's intuition. It knows what to do in most cases, but a bit of informed guidance can make the process a lot smoother. This book aims to support that natural progression, giving you the tools to understand what's happening and why, helping you make informed decisions about your care and that of your baby.

With a focus on health and wellness, the text will delve into the essentials of nutrition and safe exercise routines, designed to support your changing body and growing baby. There's a lot to consider and perhaps some habits to adjust as you 'eat for two,' with each bite a potential boost to your baby's development and your own vitality.

Moving into the second trimester, often referred to as the 'golden period,' we'll explore fetal growth and the special preparations that lay the groundwork for parenthood. From bonding with your baby to understanding developmental milestones, this stage offers a unique mix of tranquility and anticipation. Here, the emphasis is on enjoying the journey, while also starting to prepare for the reality of a new family member.

Testing and screenings are an instrumental part of any pregnancy, providing reassurance and vital insights into your baby's health. This book demystifies these processes, explaining the differences between various tests, what they can tell you, and how to interpret their outcomes with a clear and calm mindset.

Of course, pregnancy also comes with its fair share of discomforts and concerns. You'll read about navigating these challenges with practical strategies for managing symptoms and finding relief. The goal is to ensure comfort throughout your journey, allowing you to focus more on the excitement and less on the inconveniences.

Preparation is paramount as you approach the finishing line. Choosing a healthcare provider, weighing birth plan options, and considering pain management strategies are all pivotal discussions that you'll find guidance on. With each decision tailored to support your preferences and values, this book helps ease the path toward your delivery day.

The third trimester brings with it a countdown of both excitement and anticipation. We'll discuss the final mind and body preparations for labor – from understanding the early signs to knowing when it's time to head to the hospital. It's about planning for the expected while also being flexible enough to manage the unexpected.

Beyond birth, you'll find a treasure trove of resources addressing breastfeeding, newborn care, and the all-important postpartum period. These comprehensive chapters will guide you through the initial stages of nourishing and bonding with your baby, as well as taking care of yourself during recovery.

Life's complexities mean that sometimes, things don't go quite as planned. We include thoughtful considerations for high-risk pregnancies and support for those times when the unexpected occurs, ensuring you have access to compassionate advice and specialist care options, should you need them.

The conclusion of your pregnancy journey marks the beginning of yet another incredible chapter — parenthood. As you transition into this new realm, know that you've been equipped with knowledge, strengthened by support, and inspired by the countless possibilities that lie ahead for you and your family.

Let's embrace this journey together, celebrating the growth, learning from the experiences, and always remembering that at the heart of it all is the arrival of a precious new life, a unique individual who will bring their own special light into the world. Welcome to 'Expecting Joy: A Complete Guide to a Healthy Pregnancy,' your trusted guide for the incredible adventure ahead.

Chapter 2:
The Journey Begins

As we turn the page to this new chapter, we stand on the threshold of an extraordinary adventure. Embracing the whisper of life burgeoning within, we recognize the synchronization of countless miracles knitting together the fabric of a new existence. The symptoms—a missed period, a suddenly sensitive sense of smell, or an unforeseen wave of fatigue—form a tapestry of clues hinting at the profound transformation taking root. It's a time of heightened emotions; joy intertwines with anxiety as you navigate the realm of possibilities. This burgeoning chapter will guide you in interpreting the early signs, understanding the confirmation process, and the sharing of your momentous news. Through the cascade of changes, you'll find reassurance, knowledge, and the support vital to empowering your journey. With each day, as your body crafts the cradle of life, you're not just expecting—you're evolving into a testament of strength and hope, setting the stage for what's to come. Welcome to where the beauty of your journey unfolds gently—the journey begins.

Understanding Pregnancy

As we embark on this life-changing voyage together, "Understanding Pregnancy" serves as a beacon for expectant mothers and their partners, illuminating the intricate processes and profound transformations that pregnancy heralds. It is the canvas upon which nature paints the story of life's inception—an intimate journey that is as unique as it is universal. Grasping the biological symphony of conception, how a single cell evolves into a complex, heart-beating little being, is the first step in appreciating the profundity of what's occurring within. Here we explore the miraculous creation of life, from the mingling of genetic material to the establishment of the placenta, the lifeline of your developing baby. Let's nurture a deep sense of awe and respect for the incredible changes your body will experience, all while fostering a supportive environment that celebrates the strength and resilience inherent in the journey to become a parent. As we traverse each stage, from the initial realization of pregnancy to the first heartbeats and beyond, it is our privilege to offer understanding, preparing you for the chapters ahead with wisdom, empathy, and empowering knowledge.

Early Signs and Symptoms

As you embark on this beautiful, transformative journey, the very first signposts may appear subtly, almost whispering to you that a new life might be beginning within. The early signs and symptoms of pregnancy are often easy to overlook, but as you grow attuned to your body, you may begin to notice the gentle signals it sends. While every woman's experience is as unique as the life she carries, certain early signs are commonly reported and suggest it's time to take a closer look.

Perhaps one of the most well-known early symptoms is a missed period. For those with a regular menstrual cycle, this can be the first clear indicator that sparks a suspicion of pregnancy. However, some women might experience light spotting around the time their period is due, often mistaken for a light period, which can be a phenomenon known as implantation bleeding.

Tender, swollen breasts are another hallmark of early pregnancy, often arising even before a missed period. Hormonal changes are preparing your body for the journey ahead, and this can cause discomfort that feels similar to the soreness experienced premenstrually—but often, it's more pronounced.

Nausea, sometimes accompanied by vomiting, and colloquially known as morning sickness, can occur at any time of day and might creep up as early as three weeks after conception. Despite its unsettling nature, this can be seen as a reassuring sign that pregnancy hormones are in full swing, nurturing your embryo's growth.

Changes in appetite and food aversions can also signal the onset of pregnancy. You might find yourself suddenly repelled by foods you once enjoyed, or craving items you'd normally never eat. What's happening to your taste buds? These peculiar shifts are just another part of the body's natural adjustment to pregnancy.

Fatigue is another early symptom you might observe as your body begins to prioritize resources for your growing baby. You might find yourself in need of more rest or experiencing a level of exhaustion that's not typical for you. This is due to the rise in the hormone progesterone and other physiological changes that demand extra energy.

As your body keenly orchestrates the delicate process of early pregnancy, you may notice frequent urination as your kidneys adapt to increased blood flow. This can occur even before a missed period and continue throughout your pregnancy journey.

Mood swings may seem similar to the emotional upheavals sometimes experienced premenstrually, but during early pregnancy, they can intensify. The ebb and flow of hormones may send your emotions on a roller coaster ride, signaling that your body is indeed undergoing profound changes.

Heightened sense of smell is another curious phenomenon you might encounter, where previously unnoticed odors become overwhelmingly strong, further contributing to possible food aversions or nausea.

In the midst of these changes, you may also experience mild pelvic cramping or discomfort, often mistaken for the onset of a period. As your uterus begins to adjust and expand, these sensations can be amongst the very initial whispers of your growing baby.

While headaches are a common discomfort for many, an increase in frequency during early pregnancy can be caused by the surge in hormones and blood volume. It's your body's way of adjusting to the new demands placed upon it.

Constipation can also be a less-talked-about symptom of early pregnancy. The digestive system begins to slow down due to hormonal changes, emphasizing the importance of good hydration and dietary fiber.

Some expecting mothers report a metallic taste in their mouth—often described as tinged with iron—which can strike without warning. It's an odd sensation that underscores the ongoing hormonal orchestration within your body.

Lastly, while less common, a heightened basal body temperature that stays elevated can be a clue for those who regularly track their cycles. If your temperature remains high beyond the typical post-ovulation phase, it may be time to investigate further.

It's important to remember that these signs and symptoms can also be related to other factors and do not in themselves confirm a pregnancy. If you suspect you might be pregnant, a home pregnancy test can offer a preliminary answer, and follow-up with a healthcare provider can provide confirmation and guide you to the next steps in your pregnancy journey.

Listening to your body and being aware of these early signs gives you a precious opportunity to connect with your body's innate wisdom. Embrace the changes, knowing that they herald the beginning of a profound experience. As early signs blossom into a confirmed pregnancy, a new chapter filled with discoveries, challenges, and unmeasurable joy begins.

Confirming and Sharing the Good News

The moment of realizing you might be pregnant is filled with a mixture of emotions. Excitement, nervousness, and suspended disbelief all bundle together, creating a unique experience that is both personal and profound. To move from suspicion to certainty, the first step is confirming the pregnancy. Home pregnancy tests have become the initial go-to method for many, due to their convenience and quick results. Sensitivity to human chorionic gonadotropin (hCG) – the pregnancy hormone – varies among tests, so it's recommended to follow up with a healthcare provider for confirmation.

Upon receiving that positive test result, whether at home or in a more clinical setting, the journey into the boundless sea of parenthood begins. For many, the urge to share this life-changing news is powerful. However, the decision about when and with whom to share your pregnancy is deeply personal and varies for each individual and couple. Some choose to wait until the end of the first trimester when the risk of miscarriage drops significantly, while others might select a few close friends or family members to tell right away.

The manner of sharing your special announcement can range from a simple, heartfelt conversation to an elaborate reveal. These days, social media platforms are often utilized to broadcast the good news, but there's still something undeniably special about sharing the joy in a face-to-face interaction, where you can witness the emotions and reactions first-hand.

Sharing the news with a partner requires sensitivity and thought, as they're embarking on this journey with you. It's an opportunity to fortify your bond and begin embracing the upcoming changes together. It's invaluable to create a moment of connection, one where you both can express and explore your feelings openly.

For single parents or those with complex family dynamics, deciding who to tell and when can pose additional challenges. Support systems can come in many forms, and it's essential to consider who will provide the support, understanding, and excitement that this journey merits.

In the workplace, there's another layer to consider: when to tell your employer. Evaluating company policies, your role, and your comfort level with your supervisors and colleagues can guide you in deciding the timing that works to your benefit. It's important to understand your rights and the laws protecting pregnant individuals in the workplace.

An essential part of sharing your pregnancy is also preparing for others' reactions. Remember that while the news is joyous for many, it can be complex for others. Some might be dealing with fertility struggles or loss. Compassion and empathy in your approach can honor their feelings while still celebrating your own joy.

For grandparents-to-be, this revelation can be among the most endearing. Deciding whether to tell them in person, with a surprise gift, or during a family gathering can make the occasion memorable. This is a chance to deepen familial bonds and nurture intergenerational relationships.

Announcing a pregnancy to older siblings should be handled with care, keeping in mind their ability to understand and process the information. Interactive activities or books that explain the concept of a new baby can help make this transition smoother for young children.

Consideration should also go into the logistics of sharing your news. Timing is everything, and so is the setting. Choosing a quiet, comfortable environment without distractions will allow for meaningful conversation and shared emotions.

After announcing your pregnancy, you might find an outpouring of advice and stories. It's beneficial to engage with this information selectively, tapping into knowledge that feels supportive and empowering, while setting boundaries around advice that doesn't align with your values or medical guidelines.

Throughout this process, it's vital to keep your healthcare provider informed and to continue following their guidance. Regular check-ups and open communication with your provider can assure that your pregnancy is progressing healthily, giving you peace of mind while you share your news.

As you revel in the congratulations and well-wishes, it's a good idea to start thinking about your support network. This is a time to identify the people who will provide emotional and practical support throughout your pregnancy, labor, and postpartum period. These individuals will be your pillars in the incredible journey of parenthood.

Lastly, remember that everyone's experience with confirming and sharing the good news of pregnancy is unique. There are no one-size-fits-all rules for this part of the journey. It's about what feels right for you, your partner if you have one, and your growing family. Trust in your intuition, communicate with love, and allow yourself to fully embrace the joy and optimism that comes with preparing to welcome a new life into the world.

Chapter 3:
First Trimester Fundamentals

As you turn the page to the first trimester of your pregnancy, you're embarking on a profound journey of transformation that is as challenging as it is exhilarating. Your body and emotions begin an intricate dance of change, setting the stage for your little one's grand arrival. The first trimester is a period of substantial adjustment, where you'll notice physical transitions, from the oft-talked-about morning sickness to the less conspicuous shifts occurring within. It's a time when your heart may flutter with a mix of joy and apprehension, and it's perfectly natural to feel a kaleidoscope of emotions. You'll be charting a new direction in your life's map, and your prenatal visits become the waypoints that ensure you and your baby's health are meticulously monitored, offering reassurance and guidance for the journey ahead. Recognizing the fundamentals of these initial weeks helps you appreciate the silent, yet profound, whispers of life stirring inside, empowering you with knowledge and giving you the confidence to navigate this transformative era with grace and positivity.

Your Body's Changes

As you move into your first trimester, you'll soon discover that pregnancy is a time of profound transformation, not just for your baby growing inside you, but for your own body as well. Each change is a testament to the remarkable journey you are undertaking and the life you are nurturing.

The earliest transformations are often subtle. Your breasts may feel tender and swollen as they begin preparing for the vital role of feeding your newborn. This is caused by increased hormone levels, particularly estrogen and progesterone, both of which are instrumental in your pregnancy.

You may start noticing how clothes that once fitted smoothly now feel snug around your waist. A soft rounding of your lower abdomen can be one of the first physical signs that you're carrying a new life. This change occurs as your uterus starts to expand and accommodate your growing baby.

Another common change is a heightened sense of smell. This can be surprising and may result in certain fragrances you used to enjoy now evoking a strong or even nauseating response. While inconvenient, this heightened sense is believed to be your body's natural way of protecting the fetus from potentially harmful substances.

Nausea and vomiting, often referred to as 'morning sickness', can strike at any time of day and is one of the hallmarks of early pregnancy. While uncomfortable, these symptoms are typically signs of a healthy pregnancy and will usually lessen as you progress to the second trimester.

As your body adjusts to pregnancy, you might find yourself needing to urinate more frequently. This is due to your growing uterus putting pressure on your bladder. While it can be frustrating, maintaining hydration is essential for both you and your baby.

Your circulatory system is undergoing significant changes, too. Blood volume increases to support the placenta and nourish your baby, sometimes causing symptoms like dizziness or lightheadedness, especially when moving quickly from sitting to standing.

Expect some fatigue as your body works harder to support the new life inside you. It's not uncommon to feel more tired than usual, so it's important to give yourself permission to rest more and conserve energy whenever you can.

Much like the rest of you, your skin is also adapting. Some women experience the 'glow' of pregnancy, thanks to increased blood flow and oils in the skin. However, you might also notice new blemishes or skin sensitivity as your hormones fluctuate.

You may also notice changes in your hair and nails during pregnancy. Thanks to prenatal vitamins and increased hormones, your hair might feel thicker and grow faster, while your nails might grow more quickly or become harder.

Another change to be aware of is the increased likelihood of gums bleeding due to hormonal changes that can make your gum tissue more sensitive to irritation. Keeping up with dental hygiene and regular checkups is crucial during this time.

Your metabolism is getting a boost as well. You might feel a bit warmer than usual or experience hot flashes as your body works to support your baby's development; this is a normal part of the metabolic increase associated with pregnancy.

In response to all these changes, your diet and appetite may fluctuate. It's not uncommon to have cravings or aversions to certain foods. Listening to your body and discussing these changes with your healthcare provider can help you maintain a balanced diet.

Amidst these myriad of changes, your joints and ligaments will begin to loosen up in preparation for the birth process. This is thanks to a hormone named relaxin, which can lead to increased flexibility but sometimes also contributes to joint discomfort.

Finally, you might begin to experience a fluttering sensation in your lower abdomen. Known as "quickening," this can be an early sign of your baby's movements. While not everyone feels this during the first trimester, it's a subtle reminder of the new life developing within you.

These transformations are all part of your body's natural adjustment to pregnancy. They signify the extraordinary lengths your body goes to create and sustain new life. Remember to treat yourself with care, embrace the changes, and seek support when needed. This journey, with all its ebbs and flows, is as remarkable as the destination. Your body is not just changing; it's performing daily miracles.

Emotional Well-being

Embarking on the first trimester of pregnancy brings a swirl of emotions, from joy and anticipation to fear and uncertainty. It's a time when emotional well-being is as pivotal as physical health. You might find yourself riding a rollercoaster of feelings, due in part to hormonal fluctuations that are as natural as they are challenging. It's entirely normal to feel elated one moment and overwhelmed the next. Acknowledgment of these changes is the first step to harnessing inner strength. Surround yourself with a support network, find solace in the experiences of others, and don't hesitate to seek professional help if the emotional tides become too turbulent. Embrace self-care practices, whether that means quiet reflection, gentle yoga, or journaling your journey. Remember, nurturing your emotional well-being is not just about managing mood swings (a topic we delve into in a subsequent section), but about creating a strong foundation of resilience and positivity that will carry you—and your growing baby—through the rest of this transformative journey.

Coping with Mood Swings

Pregnancy can be a time of heightened emotional sensitivity, and for many, mood swings become a notable part of the experience. Understanding these emotional fluctuations and learning to manage them effectively is essential for maintaining well-being during this transformative period. While mood swings are natural, they need not dominate your pregnancy journey.

Mood swings during pregnancy can be likened to a sudden shift in the weather — clear skies followed by unexpected storms, then sun again. These swift emotional changes are often driven by hormonal fluctuations, primarily increases in progesterone and estrogen, which can affect neurotransmitters in the brain. To navigate these shifts, acknowledgment is the first step. Recognizing that mood swings are a common part of pregnancy can alleviate unnecessary worry.

Communication with your partner, family, and friends about your emotional state is vital. Transparency fosters understanding and support from your closest circles. Articulating your feelings not only aids in your own processing but also allows others the opportunity to offer the support and space you may need.

Sleep plays a crucial role in emotional health. The tiredness common in pregnancy can exacerbate moodiness, so prioritizing rest is paramount. Try to establish a consistent sleep routine, and don't hesitate to take short naps if your schedule allows. Listening to your body's need for sleep can stabilize your mood significantly.

Nutrition is another cornerstone for managing mood swings. A well-balanced diet ensures your body and brain have the necessary nutrients to function optimally. Pay close attention to your intake of Omega-3 fatty acids, as they are essential for brain health, and consider speaking with a healthcare provider about prenatal vitamins that can support emotional balance.

Regular physical activity is recommended during pregnancy, not only for your physical health but for emotional balance as well. Exercise releases endorphins, which are natural mood lifters. Whether it's a gentle walk, prenatal yoga, or another form of safe exercise, keep your body moving, as long as you have clearance from your healthcare provider.

Take the time to engage in relaxation techniques, such as deep breathing, meditation, or prenatal massage. These practices can help soothe your mind and reduce stress levels, alleviating mood swings. Classes or digital resources tailored for expectant mothers can guide you in these techniques.

Creative outlets can also serve as therapeutic tools. Journaling, painting, or crafting are activities that can distract from stress and provide a sense of accomplishment and calm. Find an activity that resonates with you and incorporate it into your routine.

Setting aside moments for connection with your growing baby can bring joy and stabilize your emotions. Simple acts, like talking or singing to your baby, can strengthen your bond and be a wonderful source of positivity and anticipation.

Remember to be gentle with yourself. Unreasonable expectations can lead to frustration and heightened mood swings. Accept that it's okay to have days when you feel less than your best — it's all part of the pregnancy process.

If mood swings become overwhelming or persistent, it's important to reach out to a healthcare professional. Sometimes mood swings can be a symptom of underlying issues, such as pregnancy-related depression or anxiety, that require professional attention.

Building a pregnancy support group, if you haven't already, can offer additional emotional reinforcement. Sharing experiences and strategies with others going through similar changes fosters a sense of community and provides a sounding board for your feelings.

Lastly, take time for reflection and mindfulness. Being present in the moment can help alleviate worries about the future and rumination on the past, offering space for emotional balance. Mindfulness can be as simple as focusing on your breath or savoring a quiet moment.

Throughout your pregnancy, remember that experiencing mood swings doesn't diminish the remarkable journey you are on. With each day, you're nurturing life and embarking on one of the most profound experiences a person can have. In the quiet and the chaos, there is beauty to be found and growth to be embraced. Trust in yourself, reach out when necessary, and celebrate each step along this extraordinary path.

Understanding mood swings as a natural consequence of the amazing process occurring within you allows for a gracious acceptance of your ever-changing emotional landscape. Layer by layer, support yourself with kindness, nourish both body and mind, and foster connections that build resilience. As you navigate these turbulent waters, the knowledge that calm seas are ahead can be the lighthouse guiding you through. Pregnancy is a singular experience, rich in both challenge and reward, and learning to cope with mood swings is a pivotal skill that not only benefits you now but is a resource for life's many journeys.

Prenatal Visits and Tests

Embarking on the beautiful journey of pregnancy, your initial prenatal check-up is your first step into a world of care tailored to ensure your health and the well-being of the little one growing inside you. Prenatal care is crucial for monitoring your pregnancy and catching potential concerns early, allowing for prompt and effective management.

Usually, the first prenatal visit happens around the 6th to 8th week of your pregnancy—right in the heart of the first trimester. You'll find this visit to be more comprehensive than the subsequent check-ups, as your healthcare provider gathers all your health information, evaluates risks, and sets the baseline for your continued care.

Detailed medical history collection is vital. You'll discuss personal health details, past pregnancies, your family's health history, and any medications you're taking. These conversations are the building blocks for personalized care and understanding any risks that might influence your pregnancy journey.

Next is a thorough physical exam. It typically includes measuring your weight and blood pressure, assessing the health of your heart, lungs, and breasts, and conducting a pelvic examination. This thorough exam provides a clearer picture of your current health status and what to expect as your body changes during pregnancy.

Blood tests are a standard part of initial screening. They're used to confirm the pregnancy's health and look for conditions that could affect you or your baby, such as anemia, HIV, and your blood type. Understanding these factors early on allows for early interventions if needed.

Urinalysis is another common test you'll encounter. It checks for urinary tract infections (UTIs), kidney problems, or diabetes. Like the blood tests, these screenings serve as preventative measures to catch issues in their earliest and most treatable stages.

One of the most anticipated moments in early prenatal visits is hearing your baby's heartbeat for the first time. This sound, often described as a rapid whooshing noise, is a powerful affirmation of the new life developing inside you. For many expectant parents, it's a profound moment laden with emotion and wonder.

An important aspect of these visits involves discussing lifestyle choices. Topics such as nutrition, exercise, and work, as well as habits like smoking or drinking, significantly impact your pregnancy. The guidance you receive here is invaluable for making informed decisions that promote a healthy gestation period.

You will also have your first ultrasound during the first trimester. This exciting peek into your womb validates the pregnancy, establishes the due date, identifies if you're carrying multiples, and ensures the baby is developing within the uterus.

Genetic screening tests will be offered to assess the risk of your baby having certain genetic disorders. These screenings are optional but can provide peace of mind or early detection for families with a history of genetic conditions.

Your healthcare provider will talk to you about proper supplementation to support your growing baby, specifically the importance of folic acid in preventing neural tube defects. This nutrient is essential in the very early stages of pregnancy, often before many women even know they're expecting.

Expect to leave your initial prenatal visit with a wealth of information and perhaps a mix of emotions. It's perfectly normal to feel overwhelmed. Take time to reflect on the information shared, and don't hesitate to reach out to your healthcare team with any follow-up questions or concerns.

Subsequent prenatal visits, which become more frequent the further you progress in your pregnancy, will monitor your baby's growth and development, as well as your health. Each visit is an opportunity to discuss any new symptoms or issues you may be experiencing. It's a safe space for your concerns and questions—a supportive environment for expecting parents to gain knowledge and reassurance.

Regular appointments are the cornerstone of prenatal care, so make them a priority. Each visit is a step toward understanding your pregnancy better and a chance to actively participate in creating a healthy environment for both you and your baby. Remember that every question you ask, every test that is run, and every piece of advice received guides you towards a safe and healthy pregnancy journey.

In partnership with your healthcare provider, you'll navigate through the complexities of pregnancy together. They're your ally in ensuring the health and safety of you and your future bundle of joy. Embrace these visits and tests—not just as medical necessities but as milestones in your pregnancy story that bring you closer to meeting your little one.

Chapter 4:
Nutrition and Wellness in Pregnancy

As we continue our journey from the initial excitement and adjustments of the first trimester, we now enter a fundamental aspect of prenatal care that sets the stage for a thriving pregnancy – nutrition and wellness. This chapter is a haven of guidance, where you'll learn that eating well isn't just about feeding two bodies; it's about nurturing two souls. We'll explore how the foods you choose impact not just your health, but the lifelong wellness of your child. Our goal is to arm you with the knowledge to make informed choices that resonate with both comfort and confidence. You'll find that the path to well-being doesn't stop at the kitchen. We emphasize the importance of staying active with safe exercise routines that not only maintain your fitness but also enhance your mental clarity and emotional balance. Remember, the journey to motherhood is a unique blend of strength and grace, and within these pages, you'll find the wisdom to embrace both. Let's embark on this chapter, where each bite and each step you take is a pledge to the bright future you're nurturing within.

Eating for Two: Nutrition Essentials

As we embark on the nourishing journey of pregnancy, the adage "eating for two" becomes a mantra for many. However, it's not just about eating more, but about eating smarter. Nutrition during pregnancy is critical, not only to support your growing baby but also to maintain your own health and prepare your body for the demands of pregnancy and motherhood.

Nutrition in pregnancy is about quality over quantity. You're nurturing a whole new life, and that requires a balance of proteins, carbohydrates, fats, vitamins, and minerals. The first essential nutrient on our list is protein. It's the building block for your baby's cells. Sources such as lean meats, poultry, fish, eggs, beans, and nuts should be part of your daily intake.

Folic acid is another cornerstone of pregnancy nutrition. It plays a significant role in reducing the risk of neural tube defects in the early stages of fetal development. Dark green leafy vegetables, nuts, beans, citrus fruits, and fortified foods are excellent sources of folic acid.

Iron is the vehicle for oxygen in the blood, and during pregnancy you need more of it as your blood volume increases. Iron-rich foods like red meat, poultry, seafood, and spinach should be paired with vitamin C-rich foods to enhance absorption. Don't forget to include a variety of fruits and vegetables in your diet to meet your vitamin C needs.

Calcium is crucial for building your baby's bones and teeth. Dairy products like milk, cheese, and yogurt are packed with calcium. If dairy isn't a part of your diet, seek out fortified plant-based milks, green leafy vegetables, and calcium-set tofu to fill the gap.

Essential fatty acids, particularly DHA, are important for brain development. Fish is an excellent source, but due to concerns over mercury, opt for choices lower in mercury such as salmon and trout, and limit your consumption to 2-3 servings a week. Alternatively, flaxseed and walnuts are good vegetarian sources.

Hydration is a key aspect of pregnancy nutrition — water carries nutrients through your body, helps digestion, and prevents urinary tract infections, which are more common during pregnancy. Aim for at least eight cups of fluids a day, and remember that fruits and vegetables also contribute to your hydration.

While this may feel like a lot to manage, remember that prenatal vitamins can act as a nutritional safety net. However, they are a supplement to a healthy diet — not a substitute. So, continue to focus on getting a variety of nutrients through whole foods.

It's important to note that some foods carry risks during pregnancy. Certain types of fish, unpasteurized dairy, and deli meats can harbor harmful bacteria. Always eat cooked fish, choose pasteurized dairy products, and if you do eat deli meats, heat them until steaming to avoid the risk of listeriosis.

Managing portion sizes and meal timing can also help with common pregnancy discomforts like heartburn and indigestion. Smaller, more frequent meals are often easier to digest and can help keep your energy levels steady.

Weight gain is a sensitive topic but is a part of a healthy pregnancy. Speak with your healthcare provider to understand how much weight gain is appropriate for your body type and pregnancy stage. Tracking your weight can help you stay within healthy guidelines, but do so with self-compassion and understanding that each body is unique.

As for cravings and aversions, it's not uncommon for these to steer your eating habits. Listen to your body, but also strive to make healthy choices. Cravings for sweets can be satisfied with fruits or yogurt instead of reaching for candy or cake. Moderation is the keyword.

When it comes to beverages, caffeine can be particularly concerning. Limiting caffeine consumption to less than 200 milligrams per day (about one 12-ounce cup of coffee) is generally considered safe. Remember to check for caffeine in sodas, teas, and even some over-the-counter medicines as well.

Finally, meal planning can be a powerful tool for ensuring a nutritious diet throughout your pregnancy. Take the time once a week to plan out your meals, emphasizing a variety of nutrient-dense foods.

Remember that each meal is an opportunity to provide your baby with the best start in life.

Now is the time to embrace your pregnant body's nutritional needs and form healthy eating habits that will last a lifetime. Nurture yourself and your baby with a balanced diet, and trust that the benefits will ripple through both of your lives. Let the joys of eating for two be not just about quantity, but about the wondrous quality of life you're cultivating with every bite.

In conclusion, while pregnancy is a time of many changes, nutrition doesn't have to be complicated. Focus on fresh, whole foods, a variety of nutrients, hydration, and safe food practices. With each healthy choice, you're supporting your baby's development and your own well-being, setting the stage for a joyful and thriving motherhood.

Safe Exercise Routines

Amid the myriad changes your body is experiencing, embracing an exercise routine that's secure for both you and your growing baby can't be overstated in its importance. It's not just about staying in shape; it's about fostering a nurturing environment for your little one right from the womb. Tailoring your physical activities to complement your pregnancy supports not only your endurance but also the robust flow of nutrients and oxygen to your baby. While intense, high-impact workouts may take a back seat during this time, many low-impact exercises like walking, prenatal yoga, and swimming can fit seamlessly into your daily regime. These activities are not merely about maintaining physical health; they also contribute significantly to your emotional resilience and overall sense of wellbeing. But remember, every pregnancy is unique, and it's crucial to consult with your healthcare provider to design an exercise plan that aligns with your body's needs and any specific medical advice you've received. As you nurture the life within, incorporating safe, doctor-approved exercises can keep you vibrant, agile, and mentally prepared for the transformative journey of motherhood.

Modifying Workouts for Pregnancy

As you adapt to the changes in your body and prepare for the beautiful journey ahead into motherhood, it's crucial to modify your exercise routine to ensure safety and effectiveness. Exercising during pregnancy can provide numerous benefits, including improved mood, better sleep, and increased stamina for labor. But not all exercises are suitable or safe during pregnancy. Let's explore how to adjust your workouts as your body and baby grow.

Firstly, it's essential to get clearance from your healthcare provider before continuing or starting any exercise regimen. Once you have the green light, listen closely to your body. Your body has innate wisdom, and it will signal when to slow down or adjust your routine to accommodate your expanding belly and shifting center of gravity.

It's recommended that you avoid high-impact exercises or activities that pose a risk of falling or abdominal injury. Instead, shift towards low-impact activities like walking, swimming, or prenatal yoga. These exercises are easier on the joints and offer the flexibility and strength-building necessary to support your changing body.

During the first trimester, you may still be able to engage in your regular exercises with slight modifications. However, as you transition into the second trimester, modifications will become more significant. Always monitor your heart rate to ensure you're not overexerting yourself—keeping it at a level where you can carry on a conversation is a good benchmark.

Strength training can still be a part of your routine, but it's wise to reduce the amount of weight and focus on higher repetitions to avoid straining. Also, consider eliminating exercises that require lying flat on your back after the first trimester, as this position can put pressure on a major vein and restrict blood flow to your heart and baby.

Core workouts are still valuable, but traditional crunches or twists may not be appropriate as your pregnancy progresses. Instead, focus on engaging your deepest abdominal muscles with gentle exercises like pelvic tilts or certain Pilates-based movements specifically designed for expectant mothers.

As your pregnancy advances into the third trimester, consider incorporating exercises that target the muscles you'll rely on during labor and delivery. Squatting and pelvic floor exercises can be particularly beneficial, helping to prepare your body for the birthing process. However, it's important to discuss the intensity and frequency of these exercises with your healthcare provider.

Hydration and rest are paramount. Always bring a water bottle to your workouts and listen to your body when it tells you it's time to rest. Pregnancy is not the time for pushing through fatigue or discomfort during exercise. Instead, it's about maintaining movement and staying healthy for both you and your baby.

It's also important to know when to stop. Watch for warning signs such as dizziness, headache, chest pain, or contractions during exercise, and cease the activity immediately if these occur. Never hesitate to contact your healthcare provider if you're unsure about a symptom or how it may affect your pregnancy.

For those who love group exercise classes, inquire if there are prenatal options available. Many fitness centers offer classes tailored to pregnant women that provide the social aspect of group exercise but are designed with the safety of both mother and child in mind.

Another consideration is apparel. Ensuring you have supportive shoes and comfortable, breathable clothing can make a significant difference in your workout experience. A good maternity sports bra and supportive belly band can provide the necessary support to keep you comfortable as your body changes.

As you near your due date, you may need to dial back the intensity and duration of your workouts significantly. This isn't giving up; it's adjusting to the physical demands of late pregnancy. You'll likely find that simple activities like walking or gentle stretching can feel like more than enough exercise during these final weeks.

Finally, remember that postpartum is also a time for adjustment. Once your baby is born, give your body the time it needs to recover before returning to your pre-pregnancy workout routine. When you do ease back into exercise, continue to be mindful of your body's signals and consider seeking guidance from a postnatal fitness specialist.

Maintaining an exercise regimen during pregnancy can be incredibly rewarding, helping to enhance not only your physical health but your emotional well-being. It empowers you with strength and resilience as you prepare to welcome your new addition. As you modify your workouts, do so with compassion and care for yourself and your growing baby, knowing that each step you take is a step towards a healthy, happy pregnancy.

Chapter 5:
Second Trimester: The Golden Period

As we turn the page into the second trimester, many of you might find a renewed zest for life coursing through your veins. It's often heralded as the 'golden period' of pregnancy for good reason—you're likely past the intense fatigue and morning sickness of the first trimester, yet still comfortably ahead of the third trimester when your growing bump becomes more of a noticeable encumbrance. During these months, your baby's development hits exciting milestones; the flutter of tiny movements signifies the burgeoning life inside you. It's also a time when many parents-to-be begin to feel more emotionally connected to their baby, as the once mystifying idea of parenthood slowly starts to crystallize into reality. Let's treasure and maximize this period by focusing on staying healthy, active, and informed without delving too deep into the specifics of upcoming prenatal tests or the aches that might arise later on. This chapter is dedicated to celebrating your pregnancy's sweet spot—the vibrant, hopeful stretch where the dream of your new family comes into sharper view.

Fetal Growth and Development

As you ease into the second trimester, often called the golden period of pregnancy, your baby's growth and development continue at an astounding pace. By now, the discomforts of the early weeks have likely diminished, and your baby, protected in the warm embrace of your womb, is quietly undertaking a remarkable transformation.

The journey of growth in these weeks is both steady and spectacular. Starting as a tiny being measuring just a few inches, your baby is preparing for significant milestones. During this time, skeletal structures harden from cartilage to bone, and a noticeable baby bump starts to show as evidence of the life burgeoning within you.

Your baby's face is becoming more defined during this period. Eyelids, which have remained closed, begin to part gradually, hinting at the first glimpses of sight. Ears are in their proper place and your baby might start responding to the sounds and voices outside, including yours. This incredible development marks the beginning of a lifelong connection between you and your child.

Delicate movements turn into kicks and somersaults as muscles strengthen. You may soon feel a gentle fluttering or a subtle nudge, a magical sensation known as 'quickening,' which is often described as one of the most memorable moments of pregnancy.

Your baby's organs continue their complex dance of growth and refinement. The heart is now divided into four functioning chambers. Meanwhile, the respiratory system is under construction with the bronchial tree fully formed, preparing your baby for that first breath of air at birth.

The digestive system matures, gearing up for its role outside your sanctuary. At this stage, your baby starts to practice swallowing by taking in amniotic fluid. This act is not just practice; it contributes to the accumulation of meconium—a collection of waste products that will be your baby's first bowel movement.

Fetal skin, initially translucent, begins to form multiple layers and is covered in a protective coating called vernix caseosa. This creamy biofilm serves as a waterproof barrier, safeguarding your baby's skin from the amniotic fluid. A fine downy hair called lanugo grows to keep your little one warm until they develop enough fat to regulate their own temperature.

With each week that passes, reproductive development progresses, determining the gender that you will soon be able to learn if you choose. The brain, already functioning and growing rapidly, lays out a complex web of neurons ensuring that, at birth, your baby will be equipped to process a barrage of new experiences.

Sensory development is also astonishing during these weeks. Taste buds appear, and the retina, responsible for processing light, develops its layers, preparing your child for the visual wonders of the world. The senses of touch and hearing are fine-tuning, setting the stage for sensory learning even before birth.

Your baby also starts a routine of sleeping and waking. Although these patterns may not match your own, rest assured, they're a sign of healthy development. You might even begin to discern a schedule as you pay close attention to your baby's active and quiet periods.

By the end of this trimester, your baby's chances of survival outside the womb have greatly increased with each week that passes. The lungs, while not fully mature, have developed to a point where they could function—with medical assistance—if a preterm birth were to happen.

Your baby is now very much resembling the infant you will soon hold in your arms, with a body that has filled out in proportion to the head. All the while, your little one grows stronger, preparing for the journey ahead. The space within your womb becomes a concert hall where each flutter feels like a greeting from the tiny person you can't wait to meet.

It's a transformative period for you as well. As your baby flourishes, you may find a newfound sense of strength and purpose. The connection between mother and child nurtures a bond that transcends the physical—it fosters an emotional and indescribable link that begins to form long before you ever gaze into each other's eyes.

Each prenatal visit reveals more about your growing baby, from ultrasound images capturing a heartbeat to the curve of a spine or the flex of a limb. These visits are not just about the measurements and medical details; they're an affirmation of the miracle developing within you.

Cherish this golden period. As your baby grows, so does the anticipation and excitement. It's a time to nurture yourself and the new life you're bringing into the world. Your journey is unique, much like the new individual taking shape and poised to add their own story to yours. Embrace it. Prepare for it. But above all, take the time to savor the incredible process that is unfolding inside you.

Preparing for Parenthood

Entering the second trimester, often labeled as the golden period, you may find yourself with a growing sense of anticipation and a tangible link to the new life inside you. Now is the ideal time to immerse yourself in preparing for parenthood—both practically and emotionally. It's a transformative journey where reading about baby development and care becomes just as crucial as reflecting on the type of parent you aspire to be. Explore different parenting philosophies, discuss expectations with your partner, and let your shared values guide the decisions you'll make. Engage in conversations about co-parenting, division of responsibilities, and aligning your family support network to ensure a collaborative approach to raising your child. Consider enrolling in parenting classes to gain confidence in handling the very real challenges of infancy and beyond. By investing time in these preparations, you're not only awaiting the birth of your child but also birthing new aspects of yourself as a nurturing caregiver, ready to embrace the responsibilities and joys of parenthood with an open heart and an empowered spirit.

Bonding with Your Baby

Now, this is a mesmerizing aspect of parenthood that begins long before your baby is born. As you navigate the journey of the second trimester, often referred to as the golden period, bonding with the little life inside you becomes an incredible part of the experience. For many, this is the time when the reality of becoming a parent truly starts to sink in.

Perhaps you've felt the first flutters, those delicate movements known as "quickening," which signal your baby's active presence. These gentle nudges are not just a sign of your baby's vitality but also an invitation to start connecting with them. Bonding involves both the heart and mind and plays a crucial role in your baby's emotional development as well as your own.

Start with something simple, like talking to your baby. The sound of your voice provides comfort and familiarity. Your baby can hear you, and responding to the sound of your voice helps to stimulate their developing brain. Share your day, read a book, or even sing – don't be surprised if you get a kick in response!

Touch is another powerful bonding tool. Gently massaging your belly can invite interaction and even help you identify your baby's sleep and wake cycles. Plus, it allows your partner to be involved and connect with the pregnancy in a tangible way. These moments can forge a deeper bond between the parents and the child before they even enter the world.

Visualizing your baby can also enhance your connection. Many find that envisioning their child helps to bridge the gap between pregnancy and parenthood. Take a moment each day to picture holding your baby, feeding them, and looking into their eyes. This mental bonding paves the way for a smooth transition once your baby arrives.

Embrace the rituals that bring you peace and a deep sense of connection. Creating a nightly routine, like playing soft music while you relax, helps not only to soothe you but also sets a pattern your baby will come to recognize and find soothing.

Never underestimate the power of your emotional wellbeing on the bonding process. Ensuring you are taking care of your mental health allows you to create a positive environment for your baby. Your emotional state is a key part of the nurturing atmosphere that encourages a strong bond.

If you have other children, involve them in bonding activities too. Encourage them to talk to the baby or to help you pick out clothes and pick names. This creates a family bonding experience, demonstrating that the arrival of a new member is a shared adventure.

Responding to your baby's kicks and movements not only acknowledges their presence but also encourages their development. Each back-and-forth interaction is like a conversation, lacking words but full of meaning and connection.

Preparing a space for your baby at home can also intensify the sense of bonding. Decorating a nursery, selecting clothes, and choosing toys are all acts that make the concept of a new baby more tangible and real.

Anticipate the moments that await you and your baby post-birth. Understanding what lies ahead, looking into breastfeeding, and learning how to care for a newborn are not just practical steps but also opportunities to mentally and emotionally prepare for the role of a lifetime.

Envisioning your first family outing, the soft cuddles after feeding, and the quiet walks in the park can be heartwarming and bonding experiences. These are the moments you will cherish and the ones worth anticipating with joy and love.

Consider practicing gentle prenatal yoga, which not only benefits your physical health but can also provide a dedicated time to focus solely on your baby. With each pose and each breath, take the time to feel your baby's presence within.

Another bonding practice is to keep a pregnancy journal, documenting your thoughts, feelings, and experiences throughout this journey. Including letters or messages to your unborn baby adds a personal touch that you can share with them in the future.

Involve your partner as much as possible. Whether it's attending prenatal appointments together or simply placing their hand on your belly to feel the baby move, these shared experiences can deepen your collective bond with the child and with each other.

Lastly, remember patience is key. Bonding is a unique and individual process that can't be rushed. It can be immediate for some, while it may take time for others. Be kind to yourself and recognize that bonding with your baby is a profound journey that takes different paths for everyone.

Embrace each of these moments, for they are the building blocks of the lifelong relationship you will have with your child. As you prepare for the chapters ahead, know that each step you take on this path is weaving the strong, loving bond that will cradle your baby from the womb into the world.

Chapter 6:
Understanding Prenatal Testing

As you stride forward into the heart of your pregnancy journey, it's essential to illuminate the role of prenatal testing—a compass for navigating the wellbeing of both you and your baby. Amid the excitement and anticipation, prenatal tests can offer reassurance and valuable insight, yet they also may bring a flutter of anxiety. These tests, varying from non-invasive screenings to diagnostic assurances, provide a means to celebrate your baby's milestones and prepare for any special care they might need. Understand that each test is a step towards safeguarding the healthy development of your child, and the choices you make about testing are deeply personal and must align with your comfort level, values, and the advice of your healthcare team. We'll demystify common tests without delving too deeply into specifics, aiming to empower you with knowledge, while reminding you of the miraculous work your body is undertaking to nurture a new life within. Rest assured, understanding what lies ahead can help transform uncertainty into confidence as you embrace this profound chapter of your life.

Screening vs. Diagnostic Tests

Advances in prenatal care offer a host of testing options that provide invaluable insights into the well-being of both mother and baby during pregnancy. But with the plethora of tests comes the need for a clear distinction between two major types: screening and diagnostic tests. The tests you will encounter, while sometimes overlapping in their

38

purpose, have distinct roles in prenatal care that are essential to understand.

Screening tests are the initial step in prenatal care - think of them as informational rather than definitive. They help to determine the likelihood of a fetus having certain genetic disorders or birth defects. The results from screening tests are typically given as probabilities or risk levels, such as '1 in 100' or 'high risk.' These tests are non-invasive and pose no risk to the fetus, making them a preferred first choice for many expectant parents.

On the other hand, diagnostic tests take a closer look when there's a possibility of a health concern, or to confirm a suspected diagnosis. Unlike screenings, diagnostic tests can usually provide a definite answer about whether the fetus has a specific genetic disorder or anomaly. However, some diagnostic tests are invasive and carry a small risk of miscarriage, which is why they are generally offered after a positive screening result or when there is a high risk of genetic conditions based on family history or other factors.

Understanding the nuances between these two test types empowers you to make informed decisions. Typical screening tests include the initial blood tests, nuchal translucency scan, and the quad screen. They serve as preliminary steps, giving you an estimate of risk without definitively diagnosing a condition.

Moving a step further, if your screening tests indicate a higher risk, your healthcare provider may suggest a diagnostic test. These tests, such as amniocentesis or chorionic villus sampling (CVS), are more conclusive because they analyze the baby's actual chromosomes.

Embarking on these tests can be an emotional process, with a mix of anticipation and anxiety. It's natural to be nervous about the results, but it's also an opportunity to embrace the support of your healthcare provider, family, and friends. They can provide the comfort and guidance needed as you navigate this comprehensive journey of prenatal testing.

While you have the choice to opt for or decline any test, making these decisions informed by the best possible information can help you feel more in control. If you choose to proceed with screening tests, you're taking a proactive step in learning about your baby's health without putting the pregnancy at risk. Should a screening result suggest further investigation, knowing that diagnostic tests are available can offer a route to clarity and peace of mind.

Never hesitate to ask questions during your prenatal visits. Your healthcare provider is there to clarify the purpose, process, benefits, and risks of each prenatal test. Seeking clarity is not only your right but also a way to ensure that you're comfortable with the path you choose for you and your baby.

For some, the choice to undergo certain tests is influenced by personal, ethical, or religious beliefs. It is a deeply personal decision whether to learn about potential challenges before birth. Honest conversations with your partner, family, and healthcare provider can help mirror your values and wishes in your prenatal care plan.

The value of screening tests lies not just in obtaining information, but in the guidance for further actions. For instance, a high-risk result doesn't necessarily mean there is a problem, but it does help to prepare for the next steps whether that is additional testing or starting conversations about what various outcomes might mean for your family.

Remember, the aim of prenatal testing is not to cause unwarranted concern but to promote a healthy pregnancy journey. Whatever the outcomes of these tests, they provide an opportunity to prepare. A prepared mind is the cornerstone of empowerment and ensures that, if needed, you'll be able to create the best care plan for your baby.

There is no one-size-fits-all approach to prenatal testing. Every pregnancy is unique, and each set of parents has their own hopes and concerns. It's a balance of embracing the joy of expecting while nurturing the life within with the utmost care and vigilance.

In the end, the choices you make about prenatal testing are highly individual, woven from your personal narrative, medical history, and the specific circumstances of your pregnancy. These choices reflect your priorities as an expectant parent, seeking health and happiness for your growing family.

As you learn about the differences between screening and diagnostic tests, take a moment to appreciate the science that makes them possible. These tests are tools designed to provide insights into your baby's development and to support you in preparing for parenthood. Regardless of which tests you choose, your journey is a shared one, with medical professionals dedicated to supporting you at every step.

While the thought of prenatal testing can be both hopeful and daunting, their purpose is clear: to pave the way for informed choices that underpin the nurturing environment you're creating for your baby. You're taking active steps in a story of care that will span a lifetime, beginning with the remarkable phase of pregnancy.

Common Tests and What They Mean for You

As you journey through pregnancy, you'll come to learn that prenatal testing is a crucial part of monitoring the health and development of your baby. These tests can provide peace of mind and valuable insights into your little one's progress. But with an array of tests available, it can be overwhelming to understand what each one entails and what the results could mean for you and your growing family.

Let's start with the basics: screening tests and diagnostic tests are two primary categories you'll encounter. Screening tests can indicate the likelihood of a problem or condition but aren't definitive; diagnostic tests provide more concrete answers. Although it's not mandatory, most healthcare providers will suggest a variety of tests at different stages of pregnancy to ensure everything is progressing normally.

One of the initial screening tests you might encounter is the **First Trimester Screening**. This combines a blood test with an ultrasound to assess the risk for chromosomal abnormalities such as Down syndrome or other genetic conditions. It's a non-invasive procedure that relies on markers found in your blood and specific measurements taken from the ultrasound.

In your second trimester, you may have the **Quad Screen**, a blood test that screens for Down syndrome, trisomy 18, and neural tube defects. While it's reassuring for most, it's important to remember that a positive result doesn't mean your baby has a condition; it simply means further testing may be recommended.

Another common and exciting test is the **Anatomy Ultrasound**, often done between 18 to 22 weeks. This comprehensive scan looks at your baby's development, checking the heart, brain, skeleton, and other critical areas. It's also when many parents get to see their baby's form more clearly, which can be a truly joyous moment.

If your pregnancy is considered high-risk or there are concerns based on screening tests, your provider might recommend a **Chorionic Villus Sampling (CVS)** or an **Amniocentesis**. Both are diagnostic tests that analyze chromosomes to detect certain genetic conditions. CVS is typically performed between 10 to 12 weeks, and amniocentesis around 15 to 20 weeks.

For women over 35 or those with a family history of certain conditions, **Non-Invasive Prenatal Testing (NIPT)** might be suggested. This blood test checks for chromosomal abnormalities and can be done as early as 10 weeks. It's highly sensitive and carries no risk to the baby, making it a popular choice.

One simple but essential test is the **Glucose Challenge Screening**, used to screen for gestational diabetes. This condition can develop during pregnancy and can affect both mother and child's health. The test usually involves drinking a sugary solution and having your blood sugar checked after an hour.

As you move closer to your due date, you may undergo a **Group B Streptococcus (GBS) screening**. GBS is a common bacterium that isn't harmful to most adults but can pose risks to newborns during delivery. Knowing your GBS status helps your medical team plan for the safest delivery possible.

In addition to these common tests, there are other specialized screenings for conditions like infectious diseases, Rh compatibility, and certain inherited disorders. Each carries its own significance and can provide crucial information for managing your pregnancy effectively.

It's important to have open conversations with your healthcare provider about each test. Understanding why they're suggested, what the potential outcomes mean, and what further steps might follow helps you feel more in control and informed throughout your pregnancy. Remember, asking questions is not only welcome, but it's also encouraged. After all, knowledge is power, and being well-informed is a step towards ensuring the best possible care for you and your little one.

While test results are usually reassuring, it's natural to feel anxious about the outcome. Each result builds a clearer picture of your baby's health, and most often, they confirm that things are progressing just as they should. However, if a test does raise a concern, rest assured that your healthcare team will guide you through the options with compassion and expertise.

Embracing the process of prenatal testing can be empowering. You are taking proactive steps towards monitoring and safeguarding the well-being of your child. In many cases, the findings from these tests can also bolster the precious bond between you and your baby, as you picture a future filled with laughter and love.

Finally, as you face these choices, remember to prioritize self-care and support. Lean on your partner, friends, family, and healthcare professionals. Your mental and emotional well-being is just as important as the physical, and support systems can be a source of immense comfort when navigating the many decisions pregnancy brings.

In summary, prenatal tests are valuable tools that serve to protect the health of both you and your baby. While some carry a degree of uncertainty, most are routine procedures that offer reassurance and critical insights. Embrace them as part of the incredible journey that you are on, and trust in the care and advice of your healthcare team. Together, you're working towards a joyful resolution – the day you get to hold your new baby in your arms.

Chapter 7:
Common Pregnancy
Concerns and Comforts

As we delve into the myriad experiences of pregnancy, it's no surprise that along with the joy comes a concoction of concerns and discomforts, each unique yet universally understood. This chapter pivots towards acknowledging the ways your body might signal its need for extra care or rest. You're navigating through a time where your lower back might protest, or your feet insist on a hiatus from those once-comfortable shoes; we're here to tackle these common pregnancy symptoms and offer pragmatic comforts. Rest assured, every twinge and niggle, from the tenderness of stretching ligaments to the snugness of jeans that pretend to fit, is heard and addressed. As you forge through this trimester, remember: your body is doing the extraordinary work of nurturing a new life, and it's doing so with remarkable resilience. Let's explore practical strategies for managing the discomforts that accompany this journey, as you equip yourself with knowledge that empowers you to embrace the ebb and flow of pregnancy with grace and confidence.

Navigating Aches and Pains

As you move through your pregnancy journey, it's not uncommon to encounter various aches and pains along the way. Your body is going through incredible transformations to accommodate the growing life inside you, and with these changes can come discomfort. It's natural to seek comfort and understanding as you navigate these physical challenges.

One of the most prevalent complaints during pregnancy is back pain. As your baby grows, your center of gravity shifts, placing additional stress on your lower back. This is often exacerbated by the softening of ligaments in your body caused by pregnancy hormones. To alleviate this discomfort, pay attention to your posture, wear supportive footwear, and consider prenatal yoga or gentle stretching exercises that can strengthen your core muscles.

Another frequent concern is pelvic pain, sometimes known as symphysis pubis dysfunction (SPD). This is due to the relaxing of ligaments preparing your body for childbirth, which can sometimes lead to misalignment or more movement of the pelvis than usual. If you're experiencing this type of pain, pelvic support belts or physiotherapy can offer relief. Avoiding activities that involve spreading your legs widely can also help manage this specific type of discomfort.

Leg cramps are another common ailment during pregnancy, particularly in the second and third trimesters. While the exact cause isn't entirely known, it's thought to be related to fatigue from carrying extra weight or changes in blood circulation. Staying hydrated and stretching your calf muscles before bedtime can help, as can ensuring you're getting enough magnesium and calcium in your diet.

Heartburn and indigestion can cause significant discomfort as your pregnancy progresses and your uterus expands, pushing on your stomach. To combat this, eat smaller, more frequent meals, avoid spicy and fatty foods, and try not to eat immediately before lying down. If these strategies don't help, consult your healthcare provider about safe antacids or medications.

Many women experience swelling, especially in the feet and ankles, as their pregnancy moves forward. This edema is caused by your body retaining more fluid and your growing uterus putting pressure on the veins returning blood from your legs to your heart. Resting with your feet elevated, staying active, and avoiding long periods of standing or sitting can lessen swelling.

Breast tenderness is often one of the first signs of pregnancy and can continue throughout, as your breasts prepare to feed your baby. Wearing a comfortable, supportive bra can ease this soreness. Look for options that have wide straps, offer good support, and are made of breathable fabric.

As your belly grows to accommodate your developing baby, you might find that round ligament pain becomes a regular part of your day. These sharp, jabbing sensations in your lower belly or groin area occur as the ligaments supporting your uterus stretch. Gentle movement, changing positions slowly, and the use of a maternity belt can provide support and relief.

Constipation and the accompanying abdominal discomfort is a common challenge during pregnancy, often due to the hormonal changes which slow down your digestive system. To help keep things moving, increase your fiber intake with whole grains, fruits, and vegetables, stay hydrated, and maintain regular physical activity as approved by your healthcare provider.

Headaches are another issue that may arise or intensify during pregnancy. They can be triggered by hormonal fluctuations, tension, dehydration, or blood sugar fluctuations. Make sure to get adequate rest, stay hydrated, manage stress, and maintain a balanced diet to help prevent or alleviate headaches.

Lastly, it's not uncommon to experience more general body aches as the weight of pregnancy takes its toll. Taking warm baths, getting massages from a professional trained in prenatal care, and practicing relaxation techniques can help soothe your tired body.

Remember that while aches and pains are a normal part of pregnancy, it's important to discuss any new or severe symptoms with your healthcare provider promptly. This is to ensure that what you're experiencing is part of the typical spectrum of pregnancy discomforts, and not a sign of something more serious.

Don't hesitate to ask for help when you need it. Whether it's seeking out a physical therapist who specializes in pregnancy care, joining a support group for expectant mothers, or simply talking to friends and family who have been through it before. Sharing your experiences and learning from others can provide comfort and practical solutions.

Keep in mind that while aches and pains are common, they do not define your pregnancy experience. Focus on the positives, like the excitement of welcoming your new child, and remember that these discomforts are temporary. Your body is performing an extraordinary feat, and it's okay to acknowledge that it isn't always easy.

Maintaining an optimistic outlook can sometimes be a challenge amidst the aches and pains of pregnancy. Yet, it's essential. Empower yourself with knowledge, support your body with gentle care, and keep your eyes on the joy that lies ahead—the arrival of your precious baby.

At every step of your pregnancy, take time to nourish your body and soul. Prioritize rest when you need it, indulge in activities that make you feel good, and always be kind to yourself as you manage the aches and pains. Each day brings you closer to holding your baby in your arms, and every challenge faced is a testament to your strength and love as a mother.

Managing Common Pregnancy Symptoms

Motherhood is a transformative journey, and each stage comes with its own set of physical transformations that can be both intriguing and challenging. Managing common pregnancy symptoms effectively is crucial for maternal comfort and well-being. As your body nurtures new life, you may find yourself facing a myriad of new sensations— from the initial waves of nausea that often signal the start of your journey, to the stretching and swelling that indicate your body's incredible adaptability. It's natural to experience symptoms like fatigue, heartburn, or changes in appetite as your pregnancy progresses. These are your body's ways of adapting to the growing demands of the little life within. Tackling these symptoms head-on with simple but effective strategies such as restful breaks, nutritional tweaks, and regular, gentle movements can be empowering. Remember, it's about finding your personal equilibrium and guiding your body through this remarkable transition. Embrace the changes and listen to your body's cues, ensuring that you provide yourself and your developing baby with the utmost care and support.

Remedies and Relief

As we navigate common pregnancy symptoms and the discomfort they may bring, it's essential to focus on remedies and relief strategies that can help you maintain comfort and well-being during this sacred time. The following guidance is crafted to support your journey, allowing you to alleviate discomfort while nurturing both your health and that of your growing baby.

During pregnancy, the body undergoes significant changes, and it's common to experience a variety of symptoms, including nausea, heartburn, and back pain. Approaching these with natural remedies and lifestyle adjustments can be incredibly effective. For instance, morning sickness can often be mitigated by eating small, frequent meals and avoiding foods that trigger discomfort.

For the many expectant mothers experiencing heartburn, small modifications can yield great benefits. Keeping meals smaller and avoiding lying down after eating can reduce symptoms. Additionally, staying away from spicy or acidic foods and wearing loose clothing can help prevent the onset of heartburn.

Back pain is another common ailment that arises as the body changes to accommodate the growing fetus. Gentle exercises like prenatal yoga or water aerobics can strengthen the muscles that support your back, providing much-needed relief. Using support pillows when sitting and sleeping can also assist in maintaining a posture that reduces strain on your back.

Leg cramps, an often-overlooked symptom, can be alleviated through stretching exercises specifically designed for pregnancy. Keeping hydrated and maintaining an intake of balanced nutrients, including calcium and magnesium, can also play a role in reducing cramps.

Swelling often affects pregnant women, particularly in the lower extremities. Elevating your feet can help, as can support stockings and ensuring you stay hydrated. Avoiding long periods of standing or sitting can also prevent fluids from accumulating in your lower limbs.

The fatigue that often accompanies pregnancy can't be ignored. Sufficient rest is crucial, so honoring your body's signals to slow down and rest is important. Incorporating short naps or rest periods throughout the day will allow you to recharge and maintain energy levels.

If you find yourself plagued by frequent headaches, staying hydrated, getting ample sleep, and managing stress are key factors in prevention and relief. A cool compress to the forehead or a gentle scalp massage can often offer immediate, albeit temporary, relief.

Constipation is a common concern due to the slow transit time in the digestive system during pregnancy. A high-fiber diet, plenty of water, and regular exercise tailored to your pregnancy can help maintain healthy bowel movements and alleviate this symptom.

Some women experience skin changes and itchiness as the belly expands and skin stretches. Keeping your skin moisturized with hypoallergenic lotions and avoiding hot showers can keep your skin hydrated and reduce itching.

Anxiety and mood swings are also prevalent due to hormonal changes and the emotional impact of pregnancy. Establishing a support network, engaging in relaxation techniques such as meditation or prenatal massage, and speaking with a healthcare professional can provide emotional relief and ensure you are getting the care you need.

Hemorrhoids can be an uncomfortable topic but are nonetheless a real concern for many. Using a sitz bath, applying witch hazel pads, and following the previously mentioned tips for combating constipation can ease discomfort and promote healing.

As the baby grows, you might encounter shortness of breath. Practicing good posture to allow maximum lung expansion and doing breathing exercises can help you cope with this symptom. It's also important to take things at a slower pace when needed.

While over-the-counter medications are available for various pregnancy symptoms, it's paramount that you consult with your healthcare provider before taking any medication to ensure safety for you and your baby. Your provider can also suggest alternative treatments that may fit your specific needs.

Lastly, prenatal vitamins are not just beneficial for baby's development; they can also help you feel your best. These supplements are designed to fill nutritional gaps and support your body as it adapts to the needs of your pregnancy.

Remember, every pregnancy is as unique as the life it nurtures. What works for one person might not work for another, and your healthcare provider is your best resource when finding remedies and relief tailored to your unique experience. Trust in your body's capacity to carry and care for your child, and take comfort in the knowledge that you have the strength and resources to meet the challenges of pregnancy with grace and ease.

Chapter 8:
Preparing for Baby's Arrival

With the nursery's palette picked and tiny clothes folded away, the calm before the baby's arrival is a mosaic of anticipation and final touches. In these moments, as you stand on the threshold of parenthood, the focus on choosing a healthcare provider crystallizes into one of the most pivotal decisions in your family's life. This choice colors the entire childbirth experience, so consider what resonates with your philosophy and hopes for your baby's birth. Simultaneously, drafting a birth plan may seem like an exercise in optimism, but it is one that ensures your preferences are voiced and understood. Delve into the myriad options and considerations with an open heart, knowing that this document is not written in stone, but rather serves as a gentle guide for the journey to come. As you weigh the importance of each preference, allow flexibility to be the underlying principle, recognizing that the ultimate goal is the health and safety of both mother and baby. Let this chapter be a reassuring hand on your shoulder, affirming that with each decision, discussion, and plan, you're taking profound steps towards welcoming your little one into a world of love and preparedness.

Choosing a Healthcare Provider

As you navigate through the chapters of pregnancy and edge closer to meeting your little one, one of the most critical decisions you'll face is choosing a healthcare provider. This professional will be your guide, confidant, and support throughout your pregnancy, labor, and delivery. When deciding on the perfect candidate to join you on this transformative journey, several considerations come into play to ensure a healthy and joyful experience.

To initiate your search, think about the type of birth experience you envision. Do you prefer a more medicalized approach, or are you inclined towards a natural childbirth? This choice will influence whether you lean towards an obstetrician-gynecologist (OB/GYN), a family practitioner, or a certified nurse-midwife (CNM) as your primary caregiver. Each provider comes with a unique perspective on pregnancy and childbirth, and knowing what aligns with your wishes is paramount.

After identifying the type of care you desire, begin researching local practitioners. Recommendations from friends and family can be invaluable, as they come with real-life testimonials to a provider's care. Online reviews and hospital affiliations of different practitioners can also offer insight into their practice and philosophy. However, remember that a decision that was right for someone else may not be the perfect fit for you.

Once you have a list of potential providers, consider their credentials and experience. Explore how long they have been practicing, the birth practices they commonly recommend, and whether they have a track record of successful, positive outcomes. Also, assess their emergency procedures and hospital affiliations to understand where you would be transferred if necessary.

The location of your healthcare provider's office and where they attend births is also crucial. Ideally, you want a location that is convenient and accessible, particularly when you are nearing your due date or in the event of an unexpected situation. Additionally, consider the hospital or birthing center's facilities, as these will be your environment during one of the most intimate experiences of your life.

It is also essential to examine the healthcare provider's communication style and availability. Frequent prenatal visits provide a glimpse into how your provider handles questions and concerns—are they patient, informative, and supportive? Open lines of communication are critical, as you should feel comfortable and respected in every interaction.

Financial considerations can't be overlooked. Discuss with the healthcare provider the costs associated with care throughout pregnancy, childbirth, and postpartum support. Ensure you have a clear understanding of what is covered by your insurance, and what out-of-pocket expenses you may incur.

During your initial meetings with a potential healthcare provider, pay attention to how they address your birth plan preferences. A responsive provider will take the time to discuss the various scenarios and choices available to you. It is vital that they respect your wishes while also providing professional insight and recommendations for the safest course of action for both you and your baby.

In certain situations, you might have specific health concerns or experience a high-risk pregnancy. In these cases, it is fundamental that your provider has the specific expertise or can refer you to specialists when required. Their ability to coordinate care with other professionals can be instrumental in ensuring the best possible outcomes for you and your baby.

Another element to weigh is the healthcare provider's philosophy on interventions during labor and delivery. Understand their standard practices and thresholds for things like labor induction, pain management, and cesarean sections. As these approaches can significantly impact your birth experience, having a provider that aligns with your preferences is key.

Throughout your pregnancy, your provider should be a source of support and education. They should facilitate access to resources such as childbirth classes, lactation consultation, and postpartum care. The commitment to your well-being should be palpable not just in the context of medical care, but in the comprehensive support they offer.

If at any point, you feel that your healthcare provider is not meeting your needs or expectations, remember it is acceptable to seek a second opinion or even change providers. While this may seem daunting, the priority is your comfort and confidence in the person who will help bring your baby into the world.

Despite the many factors to consider, trust your instincts. The rapport you build with your healthcare provider, the trust you place in them, and the mutual respect within your relationship are the cornerstones of an empowering pregnancy and birth experience. This person will witness one of the most significant moments of your life; it's essential that you feel a strong connection and trust in their expertise.

Ultimately, choosing a healthcare provider is not just about credentials and convenience. It's about finding the right partner to support you through the physical and emotional journey of pregnancy, childbirth, and beyond. When you find that provider who resonates with your values and expectations, you'll know you've taken an essential step towards a fulfilling and healthy pregnancy journey.

Welcoming a new life is a profound responsibility, and the choice of a healthcare provider is one of the first major parenting decisions you will make. Approach this choice with patience, research, and intuition, as it will set the stage for your pregnancy's narrative. With the right provider, you can look forward to an experience that is not only medically safe but also emotionally rewarding and aligned with your vision for your baby's arrival.

Birth Plans: Options and Considerations

As you approach the later stages of pregnancy, it's essential to think about your preferences for labor and delivery. A birth plan is a valuable tool that helps you articulate these preferences to your healthcare team. It encompasses choices ranging from pain relief options to who's present during the birth. While it's impossible to predict every turn your birth might take, having a plan can provide a sense of control and readiness.

A birth plan is not an itinerary set in stone but rather a set of guidelines. It communicates what's important to you and helps everyone involved understand your wishes. Be sure to discuss your birth plan with your healthcare provider ahead of time, as they can provide insights into what may or may not be feasible given your medical history and the practices at your delivering facility.

One of the first considerations for your birth plan is the setting. Would you prefer a hospital birth, a birthing center, or a home birth? Each setting offers unique benefits and potential drawbacks. Hospitals are equipped for every medical situation, whereas birthing centers offer a more homelike environment. Home births provide the comfort of familiar surroundings. Your choice will depend on your comfort level and any medical necessities.

The choice of who will deliver your baby is closely linked to where you'll give birth. Obstetricians, family physicians, and midwives are the most common options. Some expectant mothers have a strong preference for a midwife's care, which tends to be holistic and person-centered, while others feel more secure with a physician, especially if their pregnancy is high-risk.

Consideration of pain relief methods is another critical aspect of your birth plan. You have options ranging from natural techniques such as breathing exercises, hydrotherapy, and massage to medical interventions, including epidurals and analgesics. Reflect on what aligns with your philosophy and how you imagine coping with labor pain. Keep in mind that every labor experience is unique, and flexibility is crucial.

The atmosphere in the birthing room can also be a part of your plan. Some parents-to-be want dim lighting, soft music, or the presence of personal items to create a calming environment. Consider what would make you feel most relaxed and supported during labor.

Who you want by your side during delivery is a highly personal choice. Whether it's your partner, a close friend, a family member, or a doula, figure out who can best provide you with support. Remember, some delivery settings may have restrictions on the number of people allowed in the room.

Many expectant parents have preferences about interventions that might become necessary during labor. These include the use of tools such as forceps or a vacuum, or the possibility of a cesarean section. Informing yourself about these procedures and including your preferences in your birth plan can help you feel more prepared, no matter the outcome.

Your plan might also cover immediate postpartum preferences. Common considerations include whether you want to hold your baby right after delivery and if you intend to breastfeed shortly after birth. The early moments after birth can set the tone for your initial bonding experience, so think about what will be meaningful for you and your baby.

Don't forget to consider newborn procedures in your plan. Hospitals routinely perform certain actions like administering Vitamin K injections or conducting hearing tests. If you have specific wishes about when or how these procedures should be done, make them known in your birth plan.

It's important to review and revise your birth plan as your due date approaches. Your perspective might change as you learn more about the birthing process or if your medical circumstances evolve. Keep the lines of communication open with your healthcare provider to ensure your plan is still aligned with your current situation.

When creating your birth plan, focus on clarity and brevity. The goal is for any member of the healthcare team to understand your preferences quickly and easily. Use straightforward language and bullet points for easy reading.

Be realistic in your birth plan. It's vital to recognize that labor and delivery are unpredictable. Your healthcare team's primary goal will be the health and safety of you and your baby, which might necessitate deviations from the plan. View your plan as a list of preferences rather than a set of instructions that must be followed precisely.

It's also useful to think about how you'll cope if things don't go according to plan. Visualize being flexible and resilient. Equip yourself with knowledge about various birth scenarios so that you can feel empowered, rather than overwhelmed, by any changes that might arise.

Lastly, remember that a birth plan is not just a document; it's part of a broader conversation about your expectations and hopes for labor and delivery. Use your birth plan as a starting point to build trust and rapport with your healthcare team, understanding that everyone's ultimate goal is a safe and positive birth experience for you and your baby.

As you contemplate your birth plan, embrace the process with an open mind and heart. It is a wonderful exercise in envisioning the best start for your child. Consider each choice as part of the amazing journey towards parenthood, knowing your preferences are heard, respected, and woven into the tapestry of this life-changing event.

Chapter 9:
Third Trimester Countdown

As you transition into the third trimester, you've entered the home stretch of your pregnancy. It's a time filled with anticipation, as well as some natural apprehension. Your baby is growing rapidly, and you can feel that your body is preparing for the big day. You might notice Braxton Hicks contractions as your body rehearses for labor, a nesting instinct might kick in, prompting you to get your home ready for your new arrival, and with your due date inching closer, it's natural to obsess over every new twinge or sensation, wondering, "Is this it?" In this chapter, we'll focus on fine-tuning mind and body preparations for the transformative journey of labor and delivery. From recognizing true labor signs to knowing when the moment has arrived to head to the hospital, you'll gain clarity and confidence. While the finish line may seem both close and far away, trust in the strength and resilience you've cultivated throughout this journey. You're almost there, and every day brings you closer to the moment you've been waiting for—the day you meet your baby.

Mind and Body Preparations for Labor

As you embark on the final stretch of your pregnancy, your focus naturally shifts to the anticipation of labor. Preparing your mind and body for this life-changing event is an empowering journey, one that fosters resilience and readiness. A well-prepared mother approaches her labor with confidence, understanding, and a sense of calm.

Physical preparation is key. It begins with continuing the safe exercise routines you've maintained throughout your pregnancy. Exercise increases endurance – something you'll be grateful for during labor. Focus on pelvic floor exercises, which strengthen the muscles you'll rely on during the birth process. Prenatal yoga promotes flexibility and breathing techniques that prove invaluable for managing discomfort and stress.

Nourishing your body with a balanced diet also supports your body's readiness for labor. Prioritize nutrients that contribute to muscle strength and energy. Don't forget hydration; well-hydrated muscles function better, a vital aspect when those muscles need to work for hours on end.

Rest is equally essential; as your body gears up for the marathon of labor, ensuring you get adequate sleep can be beneficial. While it might be challenging to find a comfortable sleeping position, use pillows to support your body and create a restful environment to help facilitate better sleep.

Mental and emotional preparations can't be overstressed. Start with informed knowledge: understanding the stages of labor and what interventions might be necessary can help reduce fear of the unknown. Consider attending childbirth education classes to gain deeper insights and strategies for coping with labor.

Visualization and positive affirmation techniques can shape your mindset toward a positive birthing experience. Visualize yourself managing contractions successfully, and affirm your body's capability to give birth. Cultivating a positive mindset does wonders for reducing the perception of pain and anxiety.

Develop a birth plan, but hold it loosely. While it's helpful to articulate your preferences for labor and delivery, understanding that flexibility is required can help you manage expectations and reduce stress when things don't go exactly as planned.

Breathing exercises are another potent tool. Deep, rhythmic breathing not only oxygenates your body and reduces stress levels, but it also provides a focal point during contractions. Practicing various breathing techniques in advance enables you to find what works best for you.

Don't overlook the importance of emotional support. Surrounding yourself with a loving, supportive team – be they partner, family, friends, or a doula – provides comfort and encouragement. Discuss your fears and hopes with them, ensuring they know how to best support you during labor.

Journaling your thoughts and feelings can also be therapeutic as you approach labor. Putting pen to paper helps process emotions, articulate fears, and identify what you're most looking forward to once the baby arrives.

Practicing relaxation techniques such as meditation and mindfulness can help you stay present and calm. These practices also increase your pain tolerance and help in managing stress, making them invaluable during labor.

Prepare your personal space with items that soothe and comfort you. Consider a playlist of calming music, scented oils for aromatherapy, and comfy clothing that makes you feel at ease. Creating a serene environment can have a profound effect on your labor experience.

And do remember, childbirth is a uniquely personal experience. What works for one may not work for another, so it's imperative to listen to your body and trust in its inherent wisdom. Embrace the practices that resonate with you and don't hesitate to discard what doesn't serve you.

Lastly, keep the lines of communication open with your healthcare provider. Discuss your preparations and any concerns so they can provide guidance and support tailored to your needs. Their expertise is a vital resource as you prepare for labor.

As your due date nears now more than ever, nurturing your body and mind is fundamental. Honor this time with self-care and gentle attentiveness. The preparations you make now are preparations for triumph – a triumphant welcome into the world for your precious little one and for yourself, as a marvel of strength and beauty in the dance of childbirth.

Signs of Labor: When to Head to the Hospital

As you navigate the final weeks of your pregnancy, understanding the signs of labor becomes paramount. It's a time filled with excitement and anticipation, but also a time when knowing what to look for can provide both peace of mind and the readiness to act when the moment arrives. Labor can begin in several ways, and each woman's experience is unique. However, there are common signs to watch for that signal your body is preparing for childbirth.

The first and most classic sign is the onset of regular contractions. Unlike the sporadic, often painless Braxton Hicks contractions you may have been experiencing, true labor contractions are persistent, increase in intensity, and become more frequent over time. They typically last around 30 to 70 seconds and come every five to ten minutes. As time progresses, these contractions will draw closer together and won't subside with rest or hydration, as Braxton Hicks tend to do.

Another telltale sign of labor is the 'breaking of waters', or rupture of the amniotic sac. For some women, this can feel like a sudden gush of fluid, while for others, it might be a slow trickle. Amniotic fluid is usually clear or slightly pinkish in color, and it's essential to contact your healthcare provider immediately if you suspect your water has broken. This is because the risk of infection increases once the amniotic sac is no longer intact. Your healthcare team will guide you on whether you need to head straight to the hospital or wait for other signs of labor to progress.

Blood-tinged mucus discharge, known as the "bloody show," is another labor herald. This occurs as the mucus plug that blocks the cervical opening during pregnancy is discharged as the cervix begins to thin and dilate in preparation for birth. This sign can occur days before labor starts or during labor itself. Although it's a less urgent sign than contractions or water breaking, it indicates that things are moving in the right direction.

When contractions are consistent, becoming stronger, and you've noticed the bloody show or your water has broken, it's time to call your healthcare provider. They will likely ask about the timing and intensity of contractions and any other symptoms you're experiencing to help determine if it's time for you to come to the hospital.

Feeling a sudden increase in the intensity of your contractions that makes it difficult to talk through them is a sign that the labor is advancing. This is often accompanied by a strong urge to push or bear down. However, resist the urge until your healthcare provider has confirmed you are fully dilated. Arriving at the hospital before pushing is essential to ensure you and your baby are monitored and supported correctly.

If this is your first pregnancy, you might be advised to head to the hospital when contractions are about five minutes apart, lasting for a minute, and have been going on for at least an hour. However, if you've already had a baby, you may be instructed to come in sooner, as subsequent labors can be quicker.

You may also experience a significant shift in your body's physical and emotional state as you enter the early stages of labor. Emotional signs can include a burst of energy known as 'nesting,' or conversely, feelings of anxiety or irritability. Physical signs may involve diarrhea or nausea as your body clears out and prepares for delivery.

When preparing to leave for the hospital, remember to consider the logistics. If you're not in active labor yet but have signs it's imminent, it's a good time to make sure your hospital bag is packed and your transportation is ready. If you're in active labor, focus on staying calm and getting to the hospital safely.

In the event of an unexpected, rapid progression of labor—where you feel an overwhelming urge to push, see the baby's head, or experience severe bleeding—call 911 for immediate assistance. Relaying clear information to first responders can provide vital details that can guide them in offering the right support while you wait for help.

As an empowering reminder, your body has an innate wisdom and strength designed for this very purpose. Trust in your ability to recognize the signs your body is giving you. However, do not hesitate to reach out to your healthcare provider with any questions or uncertainties. It's always better to be informed and reassured than to wonder if what you're experiencing is normal.

Remember that false alarms are also possible and perfectly acceptable. If you go to the hospital and are not in active labor, don't feel discouraged. It's a common part of the journey toward childbirth, and it's always better to err on the side of caution for the well-being of you and your baby.

Finally, as you approach your due date, keep up with regular prenatal visits, as your healthcare provider will monitor signs of labor readiness, like cervical dilation and effacement. These appointments can also provide clarity on when it's time to head to the hospital based on your individual circumstances and medical history.

Your pregnancy journey is culminating in this incredible final phase. As you monitor the signs of labor diligently, remember that soon you will be holding your precious baby in your arms. Be proud of what your body has accomplished thus far, and look forward to the moment when you'll make the exciting trip to the hospital, knowing that the journey of a lifetime is about to begin—a journey of love, growth, and boundless connection with your new little one.

Chapter 10:
Breastfeeding Basics and
Newborn Care

Transitioning from the anticipatory glow of the third trimester to the profound first moments with your newborn brings a constellation of new experiences, including the essential practice of breastfeeding. This chapter gently guides you through the tender beginnings of nourishing your baby, elucidating the natural dance between mother and child that breastfeeding entails. Understanding latching techniques, recognizing feeding cues, and knowing how to gauge a successful feed can arm you with confidence as you embark on this nourishing journey. Alongside breastfeeding, we delve into the nuances of newborn care, from deciphering cries to mastering the art of swaddling, ensuring you're equipped to provide the warmth and comfort your little one needs. Meticulously curated, this chapter imparts practical wisdom on ensuring your baby's thriving growth, helping you foster an environment where love and health flourish in equal measure. Embrace these basics as the cornerstones for nurturing your newborn's early days, broadening the bond that's uniquely yours.

Preparing for Breastfeeding

Embarking on the journey of breastfeeding is akin to weaving a bond that benefits both mother and child. As we delve deeper into the chapter on *Breastfeeding Basics and Newborn Care*, it's crucial to focus on the preparation stage, which can significantly influence your breast-feeding experience.

Understanding the benefits of breastfeeding lays the groundwork for your motivation. Breast milk offers the ideal nutrition for newborns, containing a nearly perfect mix of vitamins, protein, and fat. It's more than just food; it's also packed with antibodies that help your baby fight off viruses and bacteria.

Begin by educating yourself. Attend breastfeeding classes that are often offered by hospitals or health education centers. Such classes can provide invaluable insights into the different aspects of breastfeeding, from basic techniques to recognizing and overcoming potential challenges.

Nourishment is key, not only for your growing baby but also for your own body as it prepares to produce milk. A well-balanced diet rich in fruits, vegetables, grains, proteins, and healthy fats supports milk production and maintains your energy levels.

Hydration also plays a fundamental role in breastfeeding. Drinking plenty of fluids—especially water—is essential to ensure an adequate milk supply. While there's no need to overconsume, listen to your body's thirst cues and respond accordingly.

Being comfortable can greatly impact your breastfeeding experience. Invest in supportive nursing bras and tops, which will be beneficial for easy access and comfort. Consider practicing with a breastfeeding pillow, which can help position the baby correctly and reduce strain on your arms and back.

Familiarize yourself with the concept of a proper latch, which is vital for effective breastfeeding. Seek out visual aids, such as diagrams and videos, and discuss this during prenatal visits with a lactation consultant or healthcare provider.

As you prepare, it's necessary to familiarize yourself with various breastfeeding positions. Each child and mother may find certain positions more comfortable than others, and versatility can help accommodate different situations, like feeding in public or lying down during night feeds.

Setting up a breastfeeding station at home can make the process smoother. This dedicated space can be stocked with essentials like burp cloths, water bottles, snacks, and nipple cream. Having a comfortable chair in this area with support for your back and arms is also beneficial.

Mental preparation is just as critical as the physical. Be ready to exhibit patience as both you and your newborn learn the nuances of breastfeeding. It may not be perfect from the start, but each day can bring improvement and increased confidence.

Communicating with your partner or support network about your intentions to breastfeed can ensure you have the help you might need. Discussing how your partner can be involved—whether by providing emotional support or assisting with household responsibilities—can aid in creating a breastfeeding-friendly environment.

Anticipate potential challenges that could arise, such as sore nipples or engorgement, and understand these are common and usually temporal. Knowing where to seek help, such as through a lactation consultant, can alleviate some of the stress associated with these issues.

Note the importance of self-care. While it can be easy to pour all your energy into your little one, remember that taking care of yourself through adequate rest, self-nourishment, and proper medical care is non-negotiable for both your well-being and that of your baby.

Before your baby's arrival, prepare your mindset for flexibility. While breastfeeding is the plan, sometimes adjustments must be made for the health and happiness of both mother and child. Embrace adaptability and make peace with any changes that may arise.

In the remaining sections, we will delve further into the actual act of breastfeeding, providing detailed instructions and advice for once your baby arrives. But solid preparation, as outlined here, will be essential groundwork for a successful and fulfilling breastfeeding journey.

The First Days with Your Newborn

Welcome to one of the most incredible times in your life: the first days with your newborn. Amid all the wonder and emotion, it's natural to feel overwhelmed, but remember, motherhood is a journey that begins one step at a time. In these initial days, bonding with your baby and establishing a successful breastfeeding routine are your top priorities. Let's explore the fundamental steps that will help you navigate this new and exciting phase with confidence and love.

When your newborn arrives, you'll be introduced to a delicate little person with an instinctive need to be close to you. This closeness is about more than physical contact; it's an emotional connection that begins with skin-to-skin time. Holding your baby against your skin promotes bonding, stabilizes their heart rate and temperature, and facilitates the first breastfeeding session. These quiet moments are also perfect for your partner to bond with the newest family member.

Breastfeeding might seem like the most natural thing in the world, but it's a learned skill for both you and your baby. The early days are essential for establishing your milk supply and helping your baby learn to latch properly. If breastfeeding is challenging, don't hesitate to seek help from a lactation consultant. They can offer you the support and knowledge needed to ensure both you and your child are comfortable and thriving.

You can expect your baby to feed very frequently, perhaps even every hour or two. This round-the-clock nourishment is necessary for their rapid growth and development. It's an intense time, but it won't last forever. Feeding on demand supports your infant's needs and boosts your milk production through the supply-and-demand mechanism of breastfeeding.

Diaper duty is another significant part of the first few days. Newborns may have eight or more wet diapers a day and several stools. The earliest stools, called meconium, are thick and dark but will soon pass. Their transitions to yellowish, seedy stools signify that your milk is coming in and your baby is digesting well.

Amidst the cycles of feeding and changing diapers, it's vital to look after yourself as well. You're recovering from childbirth, and your body needs rest. Enlist help from your partner or loved ones so you can take breaks, drink plenty of fluids, eat nourishing foods, and rest whenever the baby rests to replenish your strength.

Remember to keep your newborn's environment peaceful and calm. During the first days, babies are acclimating to the vastness of life outside the womb. Soft lighting, gentle sounds, and a comfortable temperature can make this transition smoother for your little one.

Babies sleep a lot during these initial days, often up to 16 hours a day, but usually in small chunks. Understanding that this intermittent sleep pattern is normal can help you set realistic expectations for your own sleep. While the nights might be long and broken, know that this phase won't last forever, and gradually, sleep patterns will evolve.

Many parents worry about their baby's breathing patterns because they can be irregular at first, varying between rapid and slow. This is typically normal as their respiratory system matures. However, if you're at all concerned about your baby's breathing, color, or behavior, don't hesitate to reach out to your healthcare provider for reassurance.

It's also time for you to learn your baby's cues. Crying is just one way infants communicate, and it can mean they're hungry, tired, need a diaper change, or simply want to be held. Responding to these cues helps your baby feel secure and loved, and teaches you to understand and meet their needs.

You'll also be adjusting to your new role and the myriad feelings that come with it. Embrace both the joy and the challenges. It's okay to feel elated one moment and exhausted the next; this does not make you any less of a loving parent.

During the hospital stay and at home, your healthcare provider will monitor your baby's weight and health. It's normal for newborns to lose some weight in the first days after birth, but they'll start gaining it back once your milk supply is established. Keeping track of weight and feedings can be reassuring to new parents and is helpful information for your pediatrician.

Embracing the support system around you is not a sign of weakness but of wisdom. Whether it's family, friends, or healthcare professionals, having support can make an immense difference in your confidence and ability to care for your newborn.

Your baby's first checkup typically occurs within the first week after birth. This visit is an opportunity to discuss any concerns you have, learn more about newborn care, and ensure everything is progressing well. It's a good time to ask questions, find out about resources, and lay the groundwork for your child's healthy development.

As you move through these first days with your new little one, trust in your abilities, and give yourself grace. You're embarking on one of the most magical and transformative journeys life has to offer. Each day with your newborn is an opportunity to grow, love, and create an everlasting bond. Cherish the moments, both big and small, and know that you are exactly what your baby needs.

Chapter 11:
Postpartum Health and Recovery

As you embark on the postpartum journey, it's important to prioritize your health and recovery with the same dedication you applied to your pregnancy. This period holds a new set of physical and emotional experiences as your body recuperates from childbirth. It's a time for healing, adjusting to new rhythms, and embracing changes with patience and care. You'll learn strategies for nurturing your body, how to recognize and manage the signs of postpartum recovery, and ways to give yourself grace during the sometimes-intense emotional transitions. Through this sensitive time, support from loved ones combined with professional advice can anchor you. This chapter is dedicated to guiding you through the postpartum period with understanding, practical tips, and a focus on holistic well-being, so you can recover with confidence and begin this next phase with strength and joy.

Physical Healing After Childbirth

Welcome to the transformative journey that continues beyond childbirth. As you step into the realm of postpartum health and recovery, the focus shifts to your own healing and well-being. The birth of a child is an extraordinary event that requires your body to undergo a series of changes as it transitions from pregnancy to postpartum recovery. Healing after childbirth is a personal and progressive journey and understanding what to expect can empower you to navigate this phase with confidence and care.

Immediately after delivery, you may experience a whirlwind of physical sensations. Your body must expel the placenta, and you will likely endure contractions, known as afterpains, as your uterus begins to contract and shrink back to its pre-pregnancy size. These uterine contractions are necessary but can be uncomfortable, especially during breastfeeding as the hormone oxytocin released can intensify these sensations.

Bleeding and discharge, medically termed 'lochia,' are normal as your body expels the remaining lining of the uterus. Initially heavy and red, this discharge will gradually lessen and change color over the next few weeks. Using heavy-duty sanitary pads during this time is advisable, as tampons can introduce bacteria and are generally not recommended until postpartum checkups confirm healing.

Whether you had a vaginal delivery or cesarean section, you will need time to recover. For vaginal births, perineal soreness is common, especially if you experienced a tear or were given an episiotomy. Sitting on cushions, using a sitz bath, and applying ice packs can alleviate discomfort, while keeping the area clean is critical for healing. If you had a C-section, caring for your incision is paramount to prevent infection and facilitate healing. Gentle movements and avoiding heavy lifting are essential while your body mends.

A common concern for many new mothers is the condition of their abdominal muscles. It's normal for the abdomen to feel loose and jiggly right after childbirth. Gentle exercise, such as pelvic tilts or deep belly breathing, can help strengthen your core muscles when you feel ready and have your healthcare provider's approval.

You may also experience swelling in your limbs due to fluid retention during pregnancy which should decrease as your body eliminates excess fluid. Elevating your feet and staying hydrated can assist in reducing this swelling more quickly.

Nursing mothers may face the challenges of engorgement, sore nipples, or mastitis. Breast care is important, so begin with proper latch techniques and don't hesitate to seek support from lactation consultants or support groups if challenges arise. Ensuring you rest and eat well can help your body produce milk and heal simultaneously.

Hemorrhoids and constipation are not uncommon postpartum concerns, often caused by the pressure of labor or reduced mobility after childbirth. A high-fiber diet, plenty of fluids, and over-the-counter remedies can provide relief; however, it's essential to consult with your healthcare provider for personalized advice.

Rest is a powerful healer, yet it can be elusive with a newborn. Sleep when your baby sleeps is sound advice not to be taken lightly. Recovery requires energy, and sleep is the best way to recharge. Balancing the demands of a newborn and your own needs is crucial. Accept offers of help with household chores to conserve your strength for healing and bonding with your baby.

Remember to listen to your body—it will signal when it's time to slow down or rest. Overexertion can hinder your recovery, and it's vital to ease back into physical activity—no matter how eager you might be to return to your pre-pregnancy routine.

Postpartum check-ups with your healthcare provider are important to ensure that your healing is on track and to discuss any concerns. These visits are ideal times to talk about birth control, breastfeeding, and how to manage any lingering symptoms you might be experiencing.

Pay attention to your nutritional needs as they play a significant role in recovery as well. A diet rich in proteins, vitamins, and minerals will support tissue repair and give you the strength you need to care for your child. Staying hydrated is also essential, especially if you're breastfeeding.

Lastly, acknowledging the emotional component of physical healing is crucial. Hormonal shifts can affect your mood and emotions, making it important to foster a supportive environment where you feel able to express your feelings and ask for help when necessary.

Everyone's postpartum recovery is unique and unfolds at its own pace. Patience with your body and grace for yourself during this transition will not only contribute to a healthier recovery but will also nurture well-being and resilience. As you gradually regain your strength, you are also growing into a new identity—a mother fortified by the journey of childbirth and endowed with the power to heal, nurture, and thrive.

Trust in the process of recovery, honor your body's pace, and celebrate the small milestones. With time, you'll find yourself embracing the new normal with energy, health, and a deeper connection to your own resilience. Embracing this chapter with both its trials and triumphs is part of the beautiful continuum of motherhood.

Emotional Adjustments and Support

The journey of motherhood does not conclude with the birth of your child; it transforms, taking on new colors and textures as you embark on the postpartum period. This chapter focuses on the crucial emotional adjustments and the relentless support that are essential during the days and weeks following childbirth.

After giving birth, you may experience a whirlwind of emotions, ranging from boundless joy to overwhelming anxiety. It's entirely normal to feel a kaleidoscope of emotions due to hormonal changes, new responsibilities, and the shift in personal identity. Navigating these feelings is a profound facet of postpartum recovery, and acknowledging them is the first stride toward emotional wellness.

One of the most common emotional developments during this time is known as the "baby blues." You might find yourself inexplicably weepy, irritable, or moody in the first few days after delivery. Bear in mind that this emotional rollercoaster is typical and, for most, short-lived, often dissipating within a couple of weeks without the need for medical intervention.

While the baby blues are transient, some new parents may encounter more intense and lasting emotional turmoil known as postpartum depression (PPD). This condition could manifest as persistent sadness, loss of interest in usual activities, or feelings of inadequacy or guilt. It's critical to seek support and professional help if these emotions become overwhelming, as PPD is a real and treatable condition.

An essential step in managing emotional fluctuations is to articulate your feelings. Speak out about your experiences with someone you trust, be it a partner, friend, or family member. Shared experiences can be incredibly validating and reassuring and can help lift the weight of isolation that sometimes accompanies the first few months of parenthood.

Remember that seeking professional support can be a sign of strength, not weakness. Therapists, counselors, and support groups offer safe spaces to delve into the complexities of postpartum emotions. These resources can give you coping strategies and connect you with others who understand what you're going through.

Moreover, self-care plays a pivotal role in emotional recovery. Prioritize rest as much as you can, eat balanced meals to support your body's healing, and carve out moments for activities that nourish your soul, whether it be a warm bath, a walk outside, or reading a few pages of a beloved book.

Also, acknowledge the magnitude of physical recovery and its impact on your emotions. The healing body can magnify feelings of vulnerability or anxiety. Respect and patience towards your body's recuperation process can have a profound effect on your mental well-being.

Bonding with your newborn can also have a therapeutic effect. Skin-to-skin contact, breastfeeding, or simply watching your baby can foster a connection and release hormones that promote happiness and love. However, if bonding doesn't happen instantly, don't be hard on yourself; like any relationship, the connection with your baby can take time to grow.

It's also beneficial to establish a rhythm to your day. While the baby's needs might determine the schedule, creating a routine can provide a sense of control and predictability, which can be incredibly soothing during a period of great change.

The role of your support network can't be overstated. Encourage your partner or family members to be involved, allowing them to take the baby for a bit to give you a breather, or seeking their help with household tasks. Here's where clear communication serves as your best ally; don't hesitate to express what you need.

Furthermore, bonding with other parents can offer a sense of community and a repository of shared knowledge and experiences. Parenting classes, online forums, or neighborhood groups can act as a lifeline, reminding you that you're not alone in your journey.

It's equally vital to monitor your progress and seek help if you notice signs that go beyond typical postpartum adjustments. If feelings of despair, detachment from your baby, or thoughts of self-harm arise, reach out to your healthcare provider immediately.

In the same vein, remember that partners can also experience emotional upheavals. Open conversation about each person's feelings and challenges encourages mutual understanding and support. This is a time to strengthen bonds and work collaboratively.

Ultimately, the postpartum period is as much about rediscovery as it is about recovery. It's a time to embrace your evolving identity and grow alongside your newborn. By weaving self-compassion, support, and understanding into your everyday life, you're building a resilient foundation for the remarkable parenthood adventure that lies ahead.

Chapter 12:
Special Considerations and Complications

In the ebb and flow of pregnancy, most journeys come with their shares of ups and downs. Yet, sometimes, you might encounter circumstances that cast a cloud of uncertainty on this special time. Whether you're facing the nuances of a high-risk pregnancy or dealing with the disheartening sense that things haven't turned out as you'd hoped, Chapter 12 is a beacon of knowledge and support. Here, you'll find heartening guidance for traversing the less-charted terrains of pregnancy that require special consideration. Remember, while certain challenges may seem daunting, being informed arms you with the strength to advocate for your health and the health of your baby. We'll explore the spectrum of potential complications without treading into the territory of diagnostics and specifics; that's the purview of your healthcare provider. But rest assured, this chapter isn't just about the 'what-ifs'—it's about fostering resilience and empowering you with the wisdom to tackle challenges with clarity and confidence.

High-Risk Pregnancies

As we venture into the realm of special considerations and complications, it's essential to understand that some journeys to parenthood may veer towards high-risk territories. A high-risk pregnancy can be an intimidating label, but with knowledge and support, it can be managed with confidence. Perhaps you're facing challenges like pre-existing medical conditions, multiple births, or pregnancy-induced health concerns; these scenarios necessitate an enhanced level of vigilance and care. It's here where teamwork takes the forefront: you'll be synchronizing with healthcare professionals who specialize in high-risk circumstances to ensure both your wellbeing and your baby's. Taking extra precautions doesn't detract from the joy of expecting; it actively protects it. The underlying message for those navigating high-risk pregnancies is to embrace empowerment through education and proactive practices, keeping your eyes on the horizon—a horizon that holds the promise of welcoming a new life, despite the storm clouds that might gather along the way.

Managing Risks and Specialist Care

As you navigate the waters of a high-risk pregnancy, it's essential to understand how to manage the risks associated with your unique situation and when you might need specialized care. High-risk pregnancies can occur for a variety of reasons, including maternal age, pre-existing health conditions, or complications that arise during pregnancy. The following guidance aims to provide you with strategies to effectively handle these risks and ensure the highest level of care for you and your baby.

First, when managing a high-risk pregnancy, communication with your healthcare provider is key. It's crucial to attend all scheduled appointments and consider seeking consultations with specialists as recommended. Depending on your situation, these may include obstetricians who specialize in high-risk pregnancies, also known as perinatologists or maternal-fetal medicine specialists, as well as other experts such as endocrinologists, cardiologists, or pediatricians with a focus on neonatology.

During these consultations, don't hesitate to ask questions and express any concerns you may have. Specialists are there to help you understand your condition and the effect it could have on your pregnancy. They can provide detailed explanations, possible treatment plans, and preventive measures to guide you through a safe pregnancy journey.

Monitoring your health and that of your developing baby is an integral part of managing a high-risk pregnancy. This may involve more frequent ultrasounds, non-stress tests, or specialized procedures like amniocentesis. Understanding the purpose of these tests and what the results mean will empower you to make informed decisions regarding your care.

Lifestyle adjustments are often recommended to cater to the needs of your high-risk pregnancy. Depending on the specifics of your condition, these adjustments could include reduced physical activity, dietary recommendations, and possibly medication to manage any underlying health issues. Always consult your healthcare provider before making any significant changes to your routine.

Although high-risk pregnancies can be stress-inducing, it's crucial to prioritize your emotional health. Strategies for stress management, such as meditation, counseling, and support groups, can promote mental wellness and indirectly benefit your baby's health. Remember that your emotional well-being is just as important as your physical condition.

In scenarios where bed rest is necessary, prepare yourself for the emotional and physical impact this can have. Make arrangements to ensure you have the support you need – whether it's help with household chores, assistance with other children, or just having someone to talk to during this time.

The risk of preterm labor is a concern that is closely monitored in high-risk pregnancies. Knowing the signs of preterm labor and when to seek immediate medical assistance can prove lifesaving. Discuss the warning signs with your healthcare provider and make sure you have a plan in place should they occur.

A delivery at a hospital equipped with a neonatal intensive care unit (NICU) may be recommended for high-risk pregnancies. If this is the case, taking a tour of the NICU and meeting with the team that may be involved in the care of your baby can alleviate some anxieties and prepare you for potential outcomes.

It's also important to be aware of and involved in decisions regarding the possible need for interventions during labor and delivery. These discussions should cover the types of interventions, the reasons they may be necessary, and how they could impact you and your baby. Knowledge is empowering and can provide comfort, even when facing the unknown.

In some cases, managing risks in a high-risk pregnancy might mean a planned cesarean delivery (C-section). If a C-section becomes a part of your birth plan, familiarize yourself with the procedure, recovery expectations, and methods to promote healing and bonding with your baby post-operation.

Medication management may also play a vital role in high-risk pregnancies. Whether it's medication to manage chronic conditions or those specific to pregnancy complications, understanding dosage, potential side effects, and interactions with other medications is essential for the safety of both you and your baby.

Nutrition and supplementation can require special attention in high-risk situations. Seek guidance from your healthcare provider or a registered dietitian to ensure that your dietary needs are being met, which may involve specific nutrient-rich foods or prescribed vitamins and supplements.

If gestational diabetes is a factor in your high-risk pregnancy, partnering with your healthcare provider to tightly control blood sugar levels through diet, exercise, and possibly medication is critical for your health and that of your baby. A proactive approach can help prevent complications related to this condition.

Finally, preparing for the possibility of an extended hospital stay, whether before or after delivery, involves ensuring that you have a support network in place. Work with your partner, family, or friends to create a plan that covers childcare, work commitments, and home maintenance so that you can focus on yourself and your newborn.

Managing risks in a high-risk pregnancy and navigating the need for specialist care can be a complex and emotionally challenging journey. Armed with knowledge, support, and a strong partnership with your healthcare team, you can move forward with confidence, advocating for the healthiest possible outcome for you and your little one.

When Things Don't Go as Planned

The journey of pregnancy can sometimes present unexpected twists and turns. While the hope is always for a smooth path to parenthood, it's important to acknowledge that not all pregnancies proceed exactly as envisioned. Preparing for the possibility of unforeseen challenges is not about fostering fear, but about fostering resilience and readiness to face whatever comes your way.

Complications during pregnancy can range from minor to more serious, and can impact both mother and baby. For some, concerns might arise early on, while for others, unpredicted issues might emerge later in the pregnancy or during delivery. These can include gestational diabetes, preeclampsia, or the baby being in a breech position, among many others.

It's crucial to maintain regular prenatal checkups, as these visits are key in early detection of potential issues. However, even with the best prenatal care, some complications can develop without warning. Learning to cope with the unpredictability requires building a strong support system, and sometimes drawing upon internal strength you may not have realized you possessed.

If a complication is detected, your healthcare provider will discuss the implications with you and outline potential courses of action. It might be overwhelming to absorb medical terminology and make critical decisions, but remember, you are never alone in the process. Don't hesitate to ask your provider to explain things as many times as you need, or to seek a second opinion if you feel it necessary.

Having a contingency plan in place can also help mitigate stress. While you may have envisioned a certain type of birth experience, being open to alternatives and understanding the reasons behind medical recommendations will help you adjust if plans need to change for the health and safety of you and your baby.

It's also helpful to educate yourself about various pregnancy complications, while keeping in mind that knowledge is power, not a reason for undue worry. Sometimes, just knowing that you are informed and on top of what's happening can make a huge difference in how you feel emotionally.

For partners and family members, witnessing a loved one experience complications can be distressing. It's important for partners to stay involved, accompany the expectant mother to appointments when possible, and offer emotional support throughout the process. Open communication within the support network ensures that everyone is on the same page and can provide the necessary support.

In some cases, it might become necessary for the mother-to-be to limit activity or even go on bed rest. Though this can be a challenging period, filled with concerns about the baby's well-being and the disruption of daily life, it is essential to focus on the positives. Use this time to connect with your baby, rest, and envision a future where both of you are thriving.

Mental and emotional health can take a hit when things don't go as planned. Reaching out to a counselor, joining a support group, or simply talking to friends and family who offer a listening ear are all valuable ways to process your feelings and find coping strategies during tough times.

Remember, there's an entire team of professionals - from obstetricians and midwives to pediatricians and nurses - ready to support and guide you. They've seen many situations and can provide the expertise and reassurance you need to navigate this part of your journey.

Amid challenges, there's often a need for difficult decision-making. This might involve considering the mode of delivery, such as a cesarean section, or making choices about the care of a premature baby. Even in such situations, your autonomy as a parent is respected, and you will play a central role in the decision-making process.

Though it's not the focus, it should be mentioned that the loss of a pregnancy, whether through miscarriage or stillbirth, is a profound and heartbreaking event some parents face. The emotional impact is significant, and those affected should give themselves permission to grieve and seek support.

Finally, it's worth celebrating every small victory and expressing gratitude for the medical interventions and support that can turn many potentially serious complications into stories of resilience and triumphant outcomes. Celebrate the strength of your body, the tenacity of your spirit, and the wonders of modern medicine. Each day brings you closer to meeting your baby, and every challenge overcome is a testament to your dedication as a parent-to-be.

While we all hope for smooth sailing, it's the storms we weather that often reveal the depth of our strength. Embrace each moment of your pregnancy journey, the expected and the unexpected, knowing that you are equipped to handle whatever comes your way. And while anticipation of the unknown can be daunting, it's the love for your child that will be your guiding light through any darkness.

In times of uncertainty, hold fast to the vision of the joy that lies ahead—the first cry, the first touch, the first gaze into your baby's eyes. These precious moments will be all the more sweet for the journey you've taken, and each challenge navigated is a step towards that ultimate joyous encounter.

Chapter 13:
The Final Stretch:
Preparing for Delivery

As you enter this concluding phase of your pregnancy, it's an exciting time filled with anticipation and preparation. You've navigated the twists and turns of pregnancy, gathering knowledge, strength, and support along the way. Now, it's about harnessing that power as you get ready for one of life's most remarkable events. In this chapter, we'll illuminate the path ahead, offering clear guidance on what to expect during labor and delivery. We understand the whirlwind of emotions that can accompany these final weeks, so we're here to provide reassurance and the tools to craft a calming birthing atmosphere. Whether exploring pain management techniques or securing your support network, remember that your body's innate wisdom and the collective knowledge of countless generations are with you. Take a moment to embrace your journey, recognizing how far you've come. And as you prepare to meet your little one, trust in the strength and love that will guide you through to that first magical embrace.

Labor and Delivery Explained

As you find yourself at the gateway of motherhood, understanding the journey through labor and delivery is paramount in fortifying your mind and embracing the process with confidence. Labor marks the culmination of your pregnancy's narrative, beginning with the first contractions and culminating in the incredible moment when you first cradle your child. It's a dynamic symphony of the body's natural rhythms and instinctual responses, comprising of well-defined stages. The initial phase is the dilation of the cervix, which sets the stage for your baby's descent. It can be both exhilarating and exhausting, as your contractions steadily work to open the path for your newborn. Transitioning then into active labor, your focus turns inwards, as breathing and relaxation techniques become vital tools. The delivery itself, the second stage, requires your deep, powerful efforts to bring your baby through the birth canal and into the world, an act as ageless as time. Finally, you'll experience the delivery of the placenta, marking the end of your labor journey. Each contraction, each breath, each moment of rest brings you closer to holding the embodiment of the love and resilience that you have nurtured for nine months.

Creating a Support System

During pregnancy, the importance of a nurturing support system cannot be overstressed. While the journey to bringing new life into the world can be a profoundly fulfilling one, it equally entails an array of challenges both physical and emotional. Designing a scaffold of support involves reaching out to those who can provide aid, understanding, and encouragement when you need it most—a cast of characters filling roles from practical helpers and sounding boards to emotional anchors.

The onset of pregnancy brings about a shared joy and excitement, as well as the need for a solid care network. Initiating conversations with family members and friends about how they can be involved is a great first step. These talks can be revelatory, helping to identify who in your circle is eager and able to step into various supportive roles during the coming months. Keep in mind that your partner, if present, will be your mainstay of support, but a diverse array of contributors can enrich this tapestry of care.

Do not underestimate the value of a healthcare provider as a part of your support system. Choose a practitioner who aligns with your values and visions for childbirth, someone you trust to guide you through every stage. Regular check-ins allow not only for medical oversight but also the fortification of a relationship that will be pivotal during childbirth. Your provider can offer peace of mind, expert advice, and a listening ear to any concerns you may have.

In the workplace, it's essential to build a network too. From discussing maternity leave policies with your human resources department to delegating tasks ahead of your leave, preparing your professional environment can alleviate stress. Colleagues who understand and support your journey can be a valuable resource, contributing to a seamless transition in and out of the workplace during this significant life event.

Community plays a critical part as well. Pregnancy support groups, either in-person or online, can connect you with others in similar circumstances. Sharing experiences and advice with fellow expectant parents can normalize the emotional rollercoaster of pregnancy and provide insider tips on managing the ups and downs. They can answer questions about their own experiences in a raw, relatable manner.

Your emotional well-being is as important as your physical health. Seeking a counselor, therapist, or joining a support group can provide an outlet for your fears, anxieties, and the inevitable stresses that come with pregnancy. A professional can equip you with coping strategies and offer a neutral perspective that friends or family might not be able to provide.

Surrounding yourself with positive influences is key. While constructive advice and shared experiences can be beneficial, every pregnancy is unique. Filtering out uninvited commentary or outdated myths that don't serve your well-being is a crucial aspect of building your network. Focus on fostering relationships with individuals who uplift and reassure rather than induce unnecessary worry or stress.

Preparing for the practicalities of a new baby is another area where a support system is invaluable. From setting up the nursery to stocking up on essentials, the tasks can be daunting. Family and friends can help you tackle the to-do lists and make the process more manageable. Even small tasks, like organizing baby clothes or preparing freezer meals, can be greatly assisted by a supportive troop.

Education is a pillar of preparation. Enrolling in childbirth and parenting classes with your partner or a support person can boost your confidence. Besides the education aspect, these courses can serve as an opportunity to meet others on the same journey, expanding your support network further.

As the pregnancy progresses and the due date nears, having a plan for who will accompany you during labor and delivery is crucial. Whether it's your partner, a family member, or a doula, this person should be someone you trust implicitly, who can advocate for your wishes, and calm you in a potentially high-stress situation. Discuss your birth plan with this person thoroughly so they understand their role and your expectations.

Doulas are an excellent addition to your support team. They offer a range of services from emotional support to educational resources, and their presence during labor and delivery can enhance the experience both for you and your partner. Their expertise in childbirth can complement the medical care provided by your healthcare team and offer reassurance during labor.

Lastly, consider a plan for after the baby arrives. Postpartum support is just as important as prenatal. Identify those who can assist with household chores, offer a listening ear as you navigate the initial stages of parenting, or simply hold the baby while you take a well-deserved rest. Ensure these individuals are aware of their roles beforehand, so they can be ready to spring into action when the time comes.

Building and nurturing your support system is a dynamic process that continues to evolve throughout your pregnancy journey. Include a mix of family, friends, professionals, and peers to address the multi-faceted needs you will encounter. Feel empowered to cultivate an atmosphere of positivity and understanding around you.

Remember, welcoming support does not compromise your independence; it enriches your resilience. Accepting help allows you to maintain your strength and focus on the miraculous task at hand—nurturing the life growing within you. Embrace the support offered, communicate your needs openly, and rest assured that by fortifying your support network, you are taking pivotal steps toward a healthy and joyful pregnancy experience.

By thoughtfully constructing a support system, you are paving a path not only to a well-supported pregnancy and delivery but to a network of relationships that can continue to flourish as your child grows. It's a profound investment in both your immediate well-being and in the fabric of a community that will surround your family for years to come.

Pain Management Options

As you approach the culmination of your pregnancy, understanding your pain management options during labor can help you feel more in control and prepared. You're embarking on a profound journey, and knowing the various ways to manage discomfort is crucial. This section is dedicated to providing insight into the array of pain relief methods available to you.

Firstly, your own body is equipped with natural mechanisms to help cope with labor pains. Deep breathing, visualization, and relaxation techniques can significantly mitigate discomfort. These methods harness the power of your mind to focus and relax your body, ultimately aiding in the natural labor process.

Beyond natural methods, medication can also play a role in pain relief. One of the most commonly used forms is an epidural, which is an anesthesia administered into the spine that dulls lower body sensation. While it can provide considerable relief, it's important to discuss the benefits and potential risks with your healthcare provider.

Another option is intravenous pain medication, which can help take the edge off contractions. While these can be effective, they don't eliminate pain entirely and may have varying effects on both mother and baby. They're typically administered in small, controlled doses to manage side effects.

It's also possible to receive a spinal block, which is given as a single injection into the spinal fluid to deliver immediate pain relief that lasts for a couple of hours. Often used during a cesarean delivery, it can be an option for vaginal births as well under certain circumstances.

For pain management without drugs, water therapy—laboring in a tub of warm water—has been praised for its soothing and pain-relieving effects. The buoyancy and warmth can help ease muscle tension and provide a calming environment.

Massage and acupressure are hands-on techniques that can help your body release endorphins—natural pain-relieving hormones. These methods can be particularly beneficial when integrated into a holistic labor plan that includes movement and positioning.

Speaking of positioning, adopting various labor positions can greatly impact your comfort levels. Simple movements like walking, squatting, and rocking can help ease pain and promote labor progress. The use of a birthing ball might also offer additional support and comfort.

Hypnobirthing is a focused method of deep relaxation, breathing, and visualization designed to reduce stress and pain during labor. By using self-hypnosis techniques, many women find they can ease their pain and have a more serene birthing experience.

For some, aromatherapy and the use of essential oils can ease anxiety and promote a sense of calm. While this method is not intended to control severe pain, it can be used as a complementary practice to create a nurturing environment.

TENS (transcutaneous electrical nerve stimulation) uses electrical pulses to stimulate nerves and reduce pain perception. A small, battery-operated device sends signals to pads on your back and is controlled by you throughout the labor process.

In addition to these options, local anesthetics or pain relief medications might be administered during repairs post-delivery if you have tears or need an episiotomy. It's typically a quick and simple process that provides immediate relief.

While discussing pain management, it's also important to be aware that plans may change. Flexibility is key, as labor can be unpredictable. It's beneficial to consider various scenarios and remain open-minded about pain relief options during childbirth.

Identifying a preferred method of pain management is deeply personal and varies from one individual to another. Equip yourself with knowledge, discuss in-depth with your healthcare team, and listen to your body. Trust that you have the strength to make informed choices that are right for you and your baby.

Please remember that there is no "right" way to manage pain during labor. Whether you opt for natural methods, medicinal aids, or a combination, what matters is that your choices align with your personal preferences and medical needs. Support from your healthcare provider, loved ones, and possibly a doula can contribute to a more positive labor experience.

Finally, as you approach the final stretch and prepare for delivery, take some time to reflect on your pain management preferences. Discuss them with your support network and incorporate them into your birth plan. By doing so, you're ensuring that your voice is heard during one of the most significant moments of your life—welcoming your child into the world.

Online Review Request for This Book

If you found "The Final Stretch: Preparing for Delivery" helpful in your pregnancy journey, please consider sharing your positive experience by leaving an online review to help others find and benefit from this resource.

Chapter 14:
Embracing the New Chapter

As the final page of this guide turns, you stand on the brink of one of life's most profound transitions. Parenthood ushers in a new chapter filled with love, growth, and unimaginable connections. This moment, the cusp of change, is both a culmination and a beginning—an embrace of the future that cradles a journey filled with joy, challenges, and discovery.

The path you've traveled—from the first flutterings of excitement to the surging waves of labor—prepares you not for a destination but for continuous transformation. Becoming a parent is not a static achievement but an evolving story resplendent with characters, narratives, and endless nuances only you can provide.

Your body's incredible metamorphosis was not solely to support life but to lay the foundation for nurturing it beyond birth. Every ache and pain, every adjustment and preparation, was part of an intricate dance that choreographed your strength and resilience. Now, as your body regains its pre-pregnancy state, recall the grace with which it adapted, and honor its journey with patience and care.

Nutrition and wellness, once meticulously managed for two, remain cornerstone elements of postpartum recovery. Your instincts, so finely tuned during pregnancy, will continue to serve as a guide. Listen to them as you balance the demands of new motherhood with the necessity of self-care.

The third trimester, with its anticipation and preparation, was but a prelude to the rhythms of parenting. The bond formed with your baby, once nestled inside, now continues in your arms, stronger and more visible with each shared gaze and touch.

Tests and screenings, previously navigated with a mix of hope and anxiety, give way to a new set of milestones and immunizations. Trust the knowledge you've gained to approach each stage with informed confidence, knowing you are equipped to make the best choices for your child.

The discomforts you managed and the remedies you discovered are now tools you'll wield with expertise, ready to soothe your newborn with a tender touch born of experience.

Baby's arrival, once an abstract concept wrapped in dreams and plans, is now a vivid reality. The choice of a healthcare provider, once a decision among many, reveals its significance as you work in partnership to ensure the health and happiness of your growing family.

Signs of labor, meticulously learned and anticipated, transform into memories that mark the beginning of parenthood. The knowledge of them now rests in the past, but the empowerment they provided continues to bolster your confidence as you navigate the myriad firsts to come.

Breastfeeding and newborn care, which once seemed like skills to be learned, are now dialogues between you and your child. Each feeding, each diaper change, is a conversation laden with intimacy and nurturing. Be gentle with yourself as you learn your baby's cues and responses, and remember that perfection lies within the patience and practice of these early days.

In postpartum health and recovery, allow the same compassion and understanding you've shown yourself throughout pregnancy to flourish. Emotional adjustments, much like physical ones, require time and support. It's okay to ask for help and essential to accept it when offered.

Should your pregnancy or delivery have included special considerations or complications, these experiences are not just chapters in your story—they're integral parts of the strength and empathy you will carry forward. From high-risk situations to unexpected outcomes, your capacity to adapt and thrive has only deepened.

As you prepared for delivery, you assembled a support system that will now shift to accommodate the dynamics of a larger family. Cherish this community, for it will be by your side through sleepless nights, celebratory milestones, and everything in between.

Pain management techniques, once a focus of your delivery plan, give way to managing the exhaustion and emotional ebb and flow of early parenthood. Your ability to weather discomfort, to find inner strength, will serve you well as you encounter the rigors of raising a child.

You've gathered wisdom, forged connections, and honed instincts that will guide you through the unpredictable landscape of parenting. Each challenge surmounted during pregnancy was not the last hurdle but a preparation for the countless acts of love and perseverance that define the role of a parent.

In embracing this new chapter, remember that while the specifics of pregnancy are behind you, the essence of what you've learned—the importance of care, education, and the boundless capacity for love— resides at the heart of parenting. Welcome to this beautiful beginning. Welcome to the incredible journey of a lifetime.

Appendix A:
Appendix

As we close this guide, full of insights and support for your pregnancy journey, we recognize that the need for information and understanding extends beyond the pages of this book. The world of pregnancy and childbirth is vast, with a myriad of resources available to you. In this Appendix, we have curated a select list of resources and support groups that can further enrich your knowledge, offer assistance, and foster a community of support during this transformative time.

Pregnancy Resources and Support Groups

Knowledge is empowering, especially when it's at your fingertips. We've assembled a collection of reputable sources to guide you through any queries or challenges you may encounter:

- **National and International Health Organizations:** These websites provide a wealth of educational materials, research updates, and health guidelines to ensure you and your baby's safety during pregnancy.

- **Local Pregnancy Centers:** These centers can offer personalized support, classes, and services tailored to your needs. They're often a hub for community connections and can bridge you to other local resources.

- **Online Communities:** Joining online forums and social media groups can link you to peers experiencing similar journeys.

Sharing stories, asking questions, and receiving emotional support in a moderated, safe space can be invaluable.

- **Maternity and Parenting Classes:** Whether it's a birthing class, breastfeeding workshop, or parenting seminar, continued education can help you feel prepared and confident as you approach labor, delivery, and beyond.

- **Hotlines:** Quick access to a knowledgeable voice can ease your worries during those moments of uncertainty. Many national hotlines are staffed by healthcare professionals ready to answer your pressing questions.

Always remember, you're not alone. If you're feeling overwhelmed, reach out. There's a community waiting to embrace you with the support and encouragement you need. Whether it's your first or third time around this miraculous journey, each experience is unique and merits its own joys, questions, and explorations.

Wishing you a healthy, empowering, and joyful progression through pregnancy to parenthood.

Pregnancy Resources and Support Groups

Entering into the journey of parenthood is one of life's most significant milestones, and it's a path best navigated with support and information. The myriad changes and decisions can be overwhelming, but rest assured, there are plentiful resources and communities designed to assist and guide you through every step of your pregnancy.

Pregnancy support groups, both in person and online, can be invaluable. They provide a space to share experiences, seek advice, and find camaraderie in the shared anticipation of parenthood. Some groups are general, welcoming anyone in the pregnancy stage, while others may focus on specific circumstances such as high-risk pregnancies or first-time parents.

Hospitals often offer prenatal classes that cover a wide range of topics from childbirth preparation to newborn care. These classes not only provide a wealth of knowledge but also introduce you to other expectant parents in your community. It's a place where you can ask healthcare professionals those burning questions and practice skills in a safe, educational environment.

Online forums and social media platforms have a plethora of groups dedicated to pregnancy and parenting. Look for those with active moderation to ensure the advice is reliable and the environment is supportive. It's a convenient way to connect with others at any time of day, which can be particularly comforting during those late-night moments of uncertainty.

For more personalized guidance, consider hiring a doula. Doulas offer emotional and physical support throughout pregnancy, childbirth, and the postpartum period. Their role complements the medical care you receive, focusing on your well-being and advocacy. They are a source of encouragement and can provide insight into the birthing process and early days of parenting.

Nonprofit organizations and charities also play a crucial role in providing resources. They can offer education, supplies, and sometimes even financial assistance to those in need. Organizations like March of Dimes and Planned Parenthood are well-established in many communities, providing specialized programs for pregnant individuals.

Books and periodicals can be a cornerstone of your learning. While there is no one-size-fits-all guide, publications written by accredited health professionals offer a wealth of knowledge. Staying informed can empower you to make the best decisions for your body and your baby.

Apps have become a modern convenience for expectant parents. Many offer week-by-week insights into fetal development, checklists, and tracking features for appointments and symptoms. Coupled with a reliable book or healthcare provider's advice, they can be a helpful tool in managing your pregnancy journey.

If you're under specific circumstances like teenage pregnancy or single parenthood, specialized support groups can offer tailored advice and a communal sense that you're not alone. They address unique challenges and celebrate the strengths necessary for these particular paths of parenthood.

Mental health resources are just as crucial as physical support systems. Pregnancy can stir a complex mix of emotions, and it's essential to have access to professionals who can help navigate these feelings. Psychotherapists, counselors, and support hotlines are options for those who need someone to talk to, particularly about topics like prenatal depression or anxiety.

Faith-based organizations often host groups that add a spiritual dimension to pregnancy support, providing comfort and guidance through shared beliefs and values. If your faith is an integral part of your life, such groups can be a cornerstone of your support system.

Don't forget that your local library can be a valuable resource. Alongside books and DVDs on pregnancy and parenting, libraries frequently host talks and workshops. They often provide bulletin boards where local resources are posted, and librarians can guide you to additional information sources.

For those interested in the latest research and insight into pregnancy health, universities and research institutions can be a goldmine. They sometimes conduct seminars or have outreach programs aimed at improving community health literacy. Staying abreast of new developments can be an enlightening part of your preparation for parenting.

Lactation consultants are there to assist with one of the initial challenges new parents face: breastfeeding. Their expertise can be invaluable both before and after the birth of your child. Many hospitals offer lactation services, but there are also independent consultants and community-based breastfeeding support groups you can join.

Lastly, remember that while resources and groups provide invaluable support, your intuition and bond with your baby are irreplaceable guides. Trust in your ability to learn and grow through this journey, and know that every question you ask, every class you attend, and every connection you make is a stepping-stone toward confident and loving parenthood.

Above all, take heart in knowing that the path you're on has been trodden by many before you, and while each experience is unique, the collective wisdom and support of a community can be the guiding light you need as you navigate the waters of expectancy and beyond.

Glossary
of Common Pregnancy Terms

As we continue through this guide, you're likely to come across terms and phrases that are specific to pregnancy and childbirth. This glossary will help demystify the language of pregnancy, so you can read with confidence and fully understand the journey you or your loved one is embarking on. Let's explore some common terms that you might encounter during pregnancy, which can provide valuable insights and clarity. Remember, knowledge is not just power—it's peace of mind.

A

- **Amenorrhea:** The absence of menstruation. In pregnancy, this is often the first sign that prompts a woman to consider she might be expecting.

- **Amniotic Fluid:** The protective liquid contained within the amniotic sac that surrounds and cushions the fetus throughout pregnancy.

- **Amniocentesis:** A prenatal test in which a small amount of amniotic fluid is sampled to check for chromosomal abnormalities and certain infections.

- **Anemia:** A condition characterized by a lower than normal number of red blood cells or hemoglobin, which can lead to fatigue and weakness during pregnancy.

B

- **Breech Position:** A fetal position where the baby's buttocks or feet are positioned to come out first during birth.

- **Braxton Hicks Contractions:** Also known as "false labor," these are irregular, usually painless contractions that may occur throughout pregnancy.

C

- **Cesarean Section (C-Section):** A surgical procedure used to deliver a baby through incisions in the abdomen and uterus.

- **Chorionic Villus Sampling (CVS):** A prenatal test involving the removal of a small piece of the placenta to check for genetic disorders.

- **Colostrum:** The first breast milk produced during pregnancy and just after birth, rich in nutrients and antibodies.

D

- **Dilation:** The opening of the cervix in preparation for childbirth, measured in centimeters from 0 (closed) to 10 (fully dilated).

E

- **Eclampsia:** A severe complication of pregnancy that causes high blood pressure and seizures.

- **Edema:** Swelling caused by excess fluid in the body's tissues, often occurring in the feet and ankles during pregnancy.

- **Embryo:** The early stage of fetal development from conception until about the eighth week of pregnancy.

- **Epidural:** A common form of pain relief during labor, where anesthesia is injected into the spinal cord area.

F

- **Fetus:** The developing baby from around the eighth week of pregnancy until birth.
- **Folic Acid:** A vital B vitamin required during pregnancy to help prevent neural tube defects in the fetus.

G

- **Gestational Age:** The age of the fetus calculated from the first day of the mother's last menstrual period.
- **Gravida:** A term used to describe the number of times a woman has been pregnant, regardless of the outcome.

H

- **HCG (Human Chorionic Gonadotropin):** A hormone produced during pregnancy that is detected in pregnancy tests.
- **Hyperemesis Gravidarum:** Severe and persistent vomiting during pregnancy that can lead to dehydration and weight loss.

I

- **Intrauterine Growth Restriction (IUGR):** A condition where the fetus is smaller than expected for the number of weeks of pregnancy.
- **Induction of Labor:** The process of using medications or other methods to start labor.

L

- **Lactation Consultant:** A professional who specializes in breastfeeding, offering support and advice to nursing mothers.

- **Lanugo:** A fine, soft hair that covers the fetus and is usually shed before birth.

M

- **Meconium:** The first stool of a newborn, a sticky, greenish-black substance that is typically passed shortly after birth.

- **Morning Sickness:** Nausea and sometimes vomiting that can occur at any time of day during pregnancy, most common in the first trimester.

Placenta:

- **Placenta:** An organ that develops in the uterus during pregnancy, providing oxygen and nutrients to the fetus and removing waste products.

- **Preterm:** Referring to a baby born before 37 weeks of pregnancy.

- **Postpartum:** The period after childbirth when the mother's body recovers and newborn care begins.

This glossary covers just a fraction of the terms you might hear on your pregnancy journey. As you navigate each chapter, keep this list at hand—it's here to support you just as much as the healthcare team and loving family around you. Stay curious, ask questions, and use this knowledge to help create a rewarding and positive pregnancy experience.

Checklists and Planners for Expectant Parents

Pregnancy is an incredible journey filled with excitement, anticipation, and, sometimes, a bit of uncertainty. As expectant parents, you have many emotions and tasks to navigate. That's where well-organized checklists and planners can come in handy. These tools will help you stay on top of everything related to your pregnancy, ensuring a smoother and more enjoyable experience. Let's dive into some practical checklists and planners to guide you through each stage of this beautiful journey.

First, let's focus on the essentials for the first trimester. The early weeks can be a whirlwind of emotions and activities. You've just learned that you're expecting, and there's so much to consider. Here's a simple checklist to get you started:

1. Schedule your first prenatal appointment.

2. Start a pregnancy journal to document your thoughts, feelings, and experiences.

3. Begin taking prenatal vitamins, including folic acid, under your healthcare provider's advice.

4. Evaluate your current medications with your healthcare provider.

5. Notify your workplace and understand maternity leave policies.

6. Cut out unhealthy habits – stop smoking and drinking alcohol.

7. Start thinking about your budget and adjusting it for baby-related expenses.

Once you've got the basics covered, it's time to concentrate on nurturing your body and mind. Pregnancy isn't just about physical changes; it's also a significant emotional journey. Using planners can help manage not just appointments, but also your diet, exercise, and overall wellness. Weekly planners can break down these areas:

Nutrition Planner:

- Weekly meal plans focusing on nutrient-rich foods.

- Grocery lists to ensure you have all ingredients for your meals.

- Hydration goals to keep you well-hydrated.

Exercise Planner:

- Customized prenatal workout schedules.

- Notes for modifying exercises as your body changes.

- Rest and relaxation days to keep you balanced and over-exertion free.

Moving into the second trimester, often known as the 'golden period' of pregnancy, you may feel more energized and less nauseous. This is a great time to prepare more extensively. Here's a checklist to make the most of this period:

- Start looking into childbirth education classes.

- Research and create a list of potential pediatricians.

- Begin setting up the nursery or baby's space in your home.

- Look into maternity clothes that are comfortable yet stylish.

- Consider making a registry for baby shower gifts.

- Plan a babymoon or a quality getaway with your partner.

During this time, both expectant mothers and fathers should think about prenatal bonding. Creating a planner for bonding activities can help you feel more connected to your baby:

- Daily or weekly time for talking and singing to the baby.

- Regular moments for your partner to feel the baby's movements.

- Parent-baby yoga or relaxation exercises.

As you enter the third trimester, the reality of your baby's imminent arrival becomes more tangible. This period calls for advanced preparation. Checklists here become crucial to ensure that you're completely ready for labor, delivery, and bringing your newborn home. Start with this comprehensive third-trimester checklist:

1. Pack your hospital bag, including essentials for you, your partner, and the baby.

2. Prepare a birth plan and discuss it with your healthcare provider.

3. Install the baby car seat and have it inspected for safety.

4. Pre-wash baby clothes, beddings, and blankets.

5. Set up a cozy and functional nursery or baby area.

6. Stock up on postpartum supplies, such as nursing pads, comfortable clothing, and sanitary pads.

7. Ensure you have all necessary documents ready for hospital admission.

The third trimester is also a wise time to think about postpartum planning. Setting up a planner for postpartum care can ease the transition after childbirth:

Postpartum Planner:

- Self-care schedule, including rest and nutritious meals.

- Feeding logs to track breastfeeding or formula feeding times and amounts.

- Appointment reminders for baby's first check-ups and your own postpartum visits.

- Daily or weekly goals to gradually resume light physical activities, only as advised by your healthcare provider.

- Contact list of friends, family, and support groups for help and emotional support.

Finally, consider the longer-term aspects of parenthood. As you wait to greet your newborn, striking a balance between planning and staying flexible is important. Here's a final checklist that may come in handy:

1. Review your insurance policies and make sure your baby will be added promptly.

2. Research and bookmark local resources for parenting and baby care, such as breastfeeding consultants, childcare providers, and parenting classes.

3. Plan for a support network, including trustworthy friends and family members who can help once the baby arrives.

4. Start thinking about your return to work or new routines if you're planning to stay home.

5. Keep a list of emergency contacts and essential phone numbers handy at all times.

Checklists and planners are indispensable tools for navigating the different stages of pregnancy and early parenthood. They not only help in managing the myriad of tasks and appointments but also provide a means to ensure you and your baby's well-being. Remember, while it's important to be prepared, it's equally crucial to embrace the journey with an open heart and mind. After all, the ultimate goal is a healthy, happy baby and well-cared-for parents ready to embark on this new chapter of life.